Ayurvedic Narcotic Medicinal Plants

Indian Medical Science Series No. 48

Ayurvedic Narcotic Medicinal Plants

Dr. C.R. Karnick
M.D, Ph.D, D.Sc, F.L.S (Lond.)

Sri Satguru Publications
A Division of
Indian Books Centre
Delhi - India

Published by:
Sri Satguru Publications
Indological and Oriental Publishers
A Division of
Indian Books Centre
40/5, Shakti Nagar,
Delhi-110007
(INDIA)

First Edition: Delhi, 1996

ISBN 81-7030-485-7

For the use only of a Registered Medical Practitioner or a Hospital or a Laboratory.

Printed in India.

Published by Sunil Gupta for Sri Satguru Publications, a division of Indian Books Centre, 40/5, Shakti Nagar, Delhi and Printed at D.K. Fine Art Press, Delhi-110 052.

Acknowledgements

The author thanks the Director, C.C.R.A.S., Ministry of Health and Family Welfare, Government of India, for continuous help during the tenure of this project.

Thanks are also due to the Director and Chairman Mr. H.F. Khorakiwala of Wockhardt Ltd., for according all facilities during the tenure of this work.

My thanks are also to Mr. Sunil Gupta of Sri Satguru Publications for taking interest and publishing this book.

Dr. C.R. Karnick
B.A.M & S., M.D.;
Ph.D. D.Sc.; F.M.S. (London)
Clinical and Experimental
Ayurvedic Research Division
Wockhardt Ltd.
Aurangabad

Contents

I

Reminiscences of Some Ancient Indian Medicinal Drug Plants

Introduction

The study of plant-life and medicine is closely related. Its genesis may be traced in various verses of the Rig-Veda which culminated in the monumental treatises of 'Charaka' and 'Susruta'. These ancient works record innumerable applications of herbs as medicines, in as much it deals exhaustively with their application in diseases and the preparation of drugs.

In the present paper the author has tried to trace the origin of some of the most important drug plants and their uses in different maladies. A special drug plant called 'Soma' - its description from ancient Hindu books is recorded.

History

All the texts of Ancient Indian Medicines have been written in verses or 'Slokas'. The first medical utterance is to be found in a text of Rig Veda in "Aushadhi Sukta" of the 10th Mandala which gives a description in details of the variety of use to which plants were put. Over hundred and seven applications are recorded. Here I quote only a few Slokas.

> "I think of the hundred and seven applications of the brown-tinted plants, which are ancient, being generated for the gods before three ages".
>
> "Mother ______(of mankind) - a hundred are your applications a thousand folds is your growth, to you who fulfil a hundred functions make this, my people free from disease".

"The `Asvavati' the `Somavati', the `Urjayanthi' the `Udojasa' (are the four principal plants) - all these I praise for the purpose of overcoming this disease".

"The plants, falling from heaven, said `The man whom living we pervade, will not perish"

(Rig Veda translation- 1907, 1-4)

"Plants, which have the Soma for your king, and who are scattered over the earth, the offsprings of Bhrishaspati, give vigour to this infirm body"

(Rig Veda VIII : 97.6)

In many hymns of Rig-Veda, we get names of certain plants with Soma, termed as the king of plants and also *Aswattha* (*Ficus religiosa* Linn, family Urticaceae) and *Palasa* (*Butea frondosa* Koeru ex Roxb., family Papilionaceae), as powerful agencies of cure against diseases.

The genesis of the whole body of medicine is given as Divine, and the nature of the cure is clearly characterised as radical permanent and comprehensive. We find that these books give a brief epitome or the germ of the science of medicine, -the art of cure, in a condensed form.

Behind the wealth of poetry one gets some facts of scientific importance. The whole thing has the air of a summary, distinctly presupposing more elaborate statements, a knowledge of details, there is no vagueness, but freshness of the original, revealed to us in an unmistakable language. Where has the details gone? They are either to all intent and purpose taken to be existence in memory (Since, it was the custom of those times that teacher showed pupils, plants in fields, but diagnostic characters and medicinal values were learnt by memory) and passed from generation to generation till they came to be synoptically recorded in some treatise and the vedic texts quoted here maybe synopsis of a synopsis.

Maladies

Their classification and remedies : Medicinal Plants are grouped in 'Atharva Veda' as follows :

1. *Kayachikitsa* (Physical maladies): those that cure physical maladies.

2. *Bhuta Vidya* (Supernatural maladies) : those that cure supernatural maladies brought about by Supernatural agencies.
3. *Kaumaravritya* (Procreation and Protection) : those that help in the procreation and protection of children.
4. *Salyavidya* (Curing wounds) : those that are used for minor and serious wounds.
5. *Vishvidya* (Cure for venom of snakes and insects) : those that are used against the venom of snakes and other insects.
6. *Rasayana* (For prosperity and prolongation of life) : those that are used for securing the prosperity and prolongation of life.
7. Vajikarana (For virility and erotic success) : those that are used for virility and erotic success.

I. Kayachikitsa

The medicinal plants of this group are mentioned in the following hymns of Atharava Veda.

(a) *For cure of leprous spots* :

"Of the bone-born leprous spot, and of the body-born that is in the skin of that made by the spoiler - by incantation have I made the white mark disappear".

(Atharava Veda I : 24.2)

(b) For becoming slim:

"The blood-drinking wizard and who so wants to take away fatness, the embryo-eating 'Kanva' do thou make disappear, O spotted leaf, and overpower".

(Atharava Veda. II. 25.39)

The plant identified is 'Mashaparni' (*Glycine labialis* family Papilionaceae) and Putta kanda (*Uraria Lagopoides* family Annonaceae).

(c) *For cure of mental diseases*.

"Born in the North, from the snowy mountain, thou art conducted to people, in the easten quarter, there they have shared out the highest name of 'Kushtha'.

(Atharva Veda V. 4.8)

"Head diseases, attack, evil of the eyes, of the body, all that may 'Kushtha' relieve, verily - a divine virility".

(Atharva Veda V. 4.10)

The plant identified is *Costus speciosus* Sm. (family-Scitaminaceae).

II. Bhuta Vidya

These are said to be due to some supernatural agencies and are mentioned in the following hymns of Atharva Veda.

(a) *Against cures*

"Let the curse go to the cursers, our part is along with him that is friendly, of the eye-conjurer, the unfriendly, we crush in the ribs." (Atharva Veda, II. 7.5)

Plant used is 'Durva' (*Cynodon dactylon* Pers. family Graminease)

"The truly-conquering, the curse-repelling, the overcoming, the reverted one, all the herbs have I called together saying - may save use from this". (Atharva Veda. IV. 17.2)

Plant used in 'Apamarga' (*Achyranthes aspera* Linn., family Amaranthaceae).

(b) *Against Ghosts or Evil Spirits*.

"The Varna, this divine forest-tree shall ward off the *Yaksha* (Ghosts), that has entered this man _____ that have the gods warded off". (Atharva Veda. VI. 85. I)

Plant used is 'Varana' (*Crataeva religiosa* Hook. family Capparidaceae).

III. Kaumaravritya

The medicinal plant of this group is mentioned in the following hymn:

"Whoever makes this woman, one having a dead child, or miscarriage, him, O, herb, do thou make disappear, lustful, for her slippery"

(Atharva Veda VIII: 6.9)

Plant used as a cure is the amulet of white and yellow mustard (*Seasamum indicum* DC. family Pedaliaceae)

IV Salyavidya

It is evident from the hymns of the Atharva Veda, dealing with the medicines for wounds, etc. that surgical treatment too was developed in Ancient India. THe following quotations will illustrate:

> "What if thee is torn, what if thee is inflamed, if crushed in thyself, may `Dhatar', excellently put that together again, joint with joint:
>
> (Atharva Veda IV. 12.2)

Plant used as cure is *Butea frondosa* Roxb. (family Papilionaceae).

> "If by a staff, if by an arrow, of if by flame, a sore is made, of O, thou art relief, relieve thou, this man".
>
> (Atharva Veda V. 5.4)
>
> "Out of the excellent `Plaksha' (*Ficus infectoria* Roxb. family Urticaceae) thou arises, out of the `Aswattha' (*Ficus religiosa* Linn., family Urticaceae), the `Khadira' (*Acacia catechu* Willd., family Mimosaceae), the `Dhawa' (*Anoqeissus latifolia* Wall., family Combretaceae), the excellent, `Nyagrodha' (*Ficus bengalensis* Linn., family Urticaceae), the parna (*Butea frondosa* Roxb. family Papilionaceae), do thou come to us, O, "Arundhati" (*Salacia* sp., family Celastraceae).
>
> (Atharva Veda. V. 5.5)
>
> "The berry, remedy for what is bruised, remedy for what is pierced, that did the gods prepare, that is sufficient for life".
>
> (Atharva Veda VI. 109.1)
>
> Plant recorded is 'Trikana' (*Piper longum* Linn., family Piperaceae),

V. Vishvidaya

It is the proud distinction of the Indian system of medicine that it has provided for the treatment against poison of snakes and insects.

The interesting fact is that the cure is not only all comprehensive and radical, but also vindictive, the agent of mischief, the snake, being compelled by virtue of remedy to take the poison of its own bite, thus the devil being hoisted with its own petard. This process might be regarded as an ancient anticipation of the modern process of autovaccination both being based on precisely the same principle of "Vishaya visha maushadham", the poison is the antidote against poison, this unqualified cure against snake-bite have been successfully practised by illiterate but skilful exorcists in obscure corners of India. The germ of snake worship as represented by the modern `Manasa Puja' maybe traced in some of the verses.

> "With sight I smite thy sight, with poison I smite thy poison, die, O, snake, do not live, let they poison go back against thee". (Atharva Veda V. 13.4)
>
> "From the cross-lined snake, from the black snake, from the adder, what is gathered - that poison of the her on jointed, one hath this plant made to disappear". (Atharva Veda VII. 56.I)
>
> The plant is 'Madhuka' (Bassia Latifolia Roxb., Sapotaceae).

VI. Rasayana

The Indian science of medicine is unique in its own way, as it deals with remedies both preventive and curative. It takes into account man, not only in a state of disease but also in a state of health. It aims both at security and the prolongation of life and in some of the hymns of the Atharva Veda, we find mention of plants which either by themselves or in association with incantations lead to longevity. Most important of these are, 'Aparajita' (*Clitoria ternatea* Linn., Papilionaceae), 'Parna' (*Butea frodosa*Roxb, Papilionaceae), 'Aswatha' (*Ficus religiosa* Linn., Urticaceae), 'Talisa' (*Flacourtia cataphracta* Roxb., Flacourtiaceae) and 'Simsapa' (*Dalbergia sissoo* Roxb., Papilionaceae).

Prosperity is sought to be brought about by the defeat of foes too, which curious as it might seem, could be brought about by the use of plants possessing supernatural properties. The plant Aparajita (*Clitoria ternatea* Linn.) is as its etymology shows, born to great invincibility and probably it is custom in Southern and Eastern parts of India, of using it as a girdle of omen around one's upper arm on the 'Bijoya' day (2nd day of Dassarah) probably it is a revival of the past practice, Quotations below carries the same meaning:

> "India put thee - (Aparajita) (*Clitoria ternatea*) on his arm, in order to allow the Asuras, smite the dispute of my counter-disputant, make them Sapless, O, herb".
>
> (Atharva Veda II, 27.3)

"Parna (*Butea frondosa*), Soma's formidable power hath come, given by Varuna, may I, shining greatly, wear it in order to length of life for a hundred autumns. (Atharva Veda III. 5.4)

"As thou, O, Aswattha d(*Ficus religiosa*) didst break out the Khadira (*Acacia catechu*) within the great sea, so do thou break out all those whom I hate, and who hate me". (Atharva Veda VI. 6.3)

VII. Vajikarana

The vital importance of the problem of virility was recognised by the Ancients in India and found remedies for increasing man's virility. The following hymns deal with these:

"I dig this herb, of plants, the strongest, with which one drives off her rival, with which one wins completely her husband".

(Atharva Veda. III. 18.I)

The plant is Vanaparni (*Clypea hernandifolia*. Menispermaceae).

"Of the horse, of the mule, of the he-goat and the ram, also of the bull, what vigorous thee are-them to thou put in him `O' self controller".

(Atharva Veda IV. 4.8)

The plant is 'Kapitthaka' (Feronia elephantum Cor., Rutaceae).

(a) SOMA

The ancient Aryans were fond of meat and drink. They used intoxicating juice of the so called "Soma plant". Rig Veda contains nearly 114 hymns on the devotional praise of "Soma", A. few verses are quoted below:

"We have drunk the same, we have become immortal.,
We have entered into light. We have known the Gods.
What can an enemy now do to us, or what can the malice of any mortal affect, O, thou immortal God?"

(Rig Veda VIII : 48.3)

"Make Vayu glad, for furtherance and bounty,
Cheer Varuna and Mitra, as they cleanse thee,
Gladden the Gods, Gladden the host of Maruts,
Make Heaven and Earth rejoice, O God, O Soma".

(Rig Veda IX : 97,42)

Virtues of Soma Juice

"The use of the (expressed juice of) Soma plant the lord of all medicinal herbs, brings about the rejuvenations of the system of its user and enables him to witness ten thousand summers on earth in the full enjoyment of a new (youthful) body. Such a person, bears a charmed life against fire, water, poison and weapon and develops a muscular energy in his limbs which would be in no way inferior to the combines strength of a thousand excited elephants of the ferocious types in their sixtieth year..... He is invested with a beauty of frame which belongs to Kandarapa (God of love) and his completion view with the beams of the full moon. The Veda with all their allied branches of knowledge instinctively drawn upon his consciousness".

(Sushruta Samhita)

Modern Aspects

Max Muller (1855) records a short botanical description, as quoted from the 'Dhutavamibhask Yatika'. He states that it is a creeper, dark in colour, sour in taste without leaves, milky, fleshy on the surface.

Watt (1890) states in his search for Soma plant that he was able to obtain a sample of 'Soma' from Bombay and the sample was identical to *Periploca aphylla* which is an erect, leafless perennial shrub with twings thicker as goose-quill. The plant possesses milky sap. Here I quote the description of 'Soma' plant as given in Sushruta Samhita:

"A Soma plant of whatever species (24 varieties), is furnished with 15 leaves which waxes and wanes with the phases of moon. Thus one leaf grows every day in the lighted fortnight attaining the greatest number (15) in the night of full moon and then the leaves begin to decrease in number dropping one by one till the bare stem of the creeper is left on the night of the new moon".

"The amsuman species of the Soma is characterised by a smell like that of clarified butter and has a bulb, while the Rajataprabha is possessed of a bulb resembling a plantain in shape. The Munjavan puts forth leaves like those of a garlic while the Chandramah species is possessed of a golden colour and is aquatic in its habitat. The Garudahrita and Svetaksha species are yellow (Pandura) and looks like the cast of skin of a snake and are usually found to be pendent from the boughs of the trees".

Probable species

Vedic description of Soma specie	*Probable botanical identity*
Smsuman species of Soma characterised with smell of clarified butter and has bulb.	i) *Ceropeqia bulbosa.* ii) *Dioscorea bulbifera.* iii) *Ceropeqia rollae.*
Rajataprabha species of Soma possesses a bulb and resembling a plantain in shape.	i) *Ceropeqia tuberosa* with tuberous root. ii) *Dioscorea esculenta* which has rhisome like plantain.
Munjavan species of Soma puts forth leaves like those of garlic.	i) *Sacrostemma brevestiqma.*
Chandramah species of Soma is possessed of golden colour and aquatic in habitat.	i) *Periploca qraeca,* hygrophyte from Mediterranean.
Garudahrita and Svetaksha species of Soma, looks like a "Cast of skin of snake".	i) *Dioscorea bulbifera* with bulb and the stem shows outer epidermis like skin of snake.

References

Charaka: English translation by Abinash Ch. Kaviratna Fasc. II. XI, XII, XIII, XXIII, XXIV and LXI, 1928.

Clayton A.D. The Rig-Veda and Vedic Religion Christian Literature Society for India, London 1:292, 1913.

Ganapathy C.V. and Sastry B.N. Current Sci. *9*, 413, 1940. Griffth. R.T. The Hymns of the Rig-Veda. Benares. Max Muller. India: What can it teach us. Longmans. 1883. Max Muller: Ancient Sanskrit Literature, 1884. Wilson, J. India, three thousand years ago, Bombay 1907. Wilson, H.H. Translation of the *Rigveda Samhita* Allen & Co. 1907. Whitney I. English translation of Atharava Veda 1908.

II

SOMA

Rig-Vedas, is one of the oldest repositories of human knowledge. Exact date of origin, is still in antiquity, but is is said to have been written some-where between 2,000 and 2,500 B.C. even earlier some-where in the third millennium B.C.[2]

Indian Sub-continent was then under a thick cover of temperate forest zones, and sheets of ice-belts were shifting in the north, while the sub-tropical vain forests abounded in the larger positions of the peninsula. The land-mass probably was then in the shadow of heavy precipitation.

This study begins during third millennium B.C. (1) Probably there was a massive and gradual shifting of ice-ages[3] from the Siberian continent to the Southern flanks of Himalayas (c.f. Plate I).

Aryan tribes from Siberian hinterland migrated south-wards, via Iran through Himalayan passes (Bolan and Khyber) into the Northern parts of India.

A great Indo-Aryan civilisation, then flourished on the fertile plains of River Indus, Ganges and its tributaries. Much has been forgotten about the Saraswati,[4] (a tributary of river Indus) which flowed from Sirmur into the plains of Abdari (Additirtha)., the present day flat-lands of Rajasthan.

The Aryans were so advanced in their technological developments, that they generally used special type of chariots which could traverse high and low-lands with ease, not unlike the present day helicopters(!), very frequently they travelled to and fro from the Siberian hinterlands, then termed as the "Rajika country" which was situated to the extreme north of the Himalayas. Further north, in the Siberian plains occur a lake often referred to as `Baykal lake' where the so-called `Sharyat' hamlets abounded.

We will now scan the pages of Rig-Vedas and quote the different stanzas, from various Mandalas, especially VIII and IX to get the clear picture of the plant in question (i.e. "Soma-plant").

1. Locality

VIII_2^{-29} सुबोमे शर्यणावत्यार्जिके नस्त्यावति ।
वयुनिचक्रया नरः ।। २९ ।।

The leaders of rites have proceeded with down-ward chariots to the Rijika country, while lies the Sharyanavat abounding in dwellings, and where soma is plentiful29.

2. Description

$IX\text{-}_{10}^{29}$ अभि प्रिया दिवस्नदमध्वर्युभिर्गुहा हितम् ।
सुरः पश्यति चक्षसा ।। ९ ।।

O' (Soma), anoint with the streaming honey-God Vanaspati, shining, yellow-coloured golden-coloured ।।10।।

The sun when seen at twilights or at dawn shows an appearance no unlike of a flaming yellowish-red or golden coloured disk., this colour is attributed to Soma.

IX_2^6 अचि क्रदद् वृषा हरिर्महान् मित्रो न दर्शतः ।
सं सूर्येण रोचते ।। ६ ।।

(Soma), who produces a sound, the showerer of desire, of tawny-colour, the best of all, worthy of seeing, like a friend shines with sun ।।6।।

Soma-plant is of a reddish-brown colour, compared with shining disc of sun which is orange-red in colour.

Further the growth stages of plant has been simulated with stages of rising sun-

IX_{64}^8 केतु कृण्वन दिवस्परी विश्रवा रुपाभ्यर्षसि ।
समुद्रः सोम पिन्वसे ।। ८ ।।

IX_{64}^9 हिन्वानो वाचमिष्यसि पवमान वर्धमाणि ।
अक्रान देवो न सूर्याः ।। ९ ।।

Being urged onwards, sendest upO, Pavvamana, in order to spread out, thou hast stridden liken the sun 9 The plant is distinguished into a upper region, the (middle) portion, the stalk which rises from the wet moulds of earth. The cap of the (mushroom) increases in size, simultaneously becoming bright red to orange red on colour as it grows. This has been compared with the stage so rising sun.

IX_{61}^{21} समिश्रलो अरुषो भव सूपस्थाभिर्न धेनुभि।
सदिञ्छयेनो न योनिमा ।। २१ ।।

Mixed, become red in the company of "ample-hipped" cows, sitting on, seat like a faleon" ||21||

Soma-plant becomes bright-red in colour & appears to sits like an eagle.

VIII_3^5 इन्द्रमिद् देवतातय इन्द्रं प्रयत्यध्वरे।
इन्द्रं समीके वनिनो हवामह इन्द्रं धनस्य सातये।। ५।।

May this soma, invested, approach these.

observant Indra, like a bride clad in white apparel ||5||

With the expansion of the mushroom cap, it attains white flecks these cover underlying red skin of the mushroom, figuratively appears not unlike a bride in white dress (!)

IX_{97}^9 सं रहत उरुगायस्य जूति वृथा क्रीळन्तं मिमते नगावः।
परीणसं कृणुते तिग्मशृङ्गो दिवा हरिर्दहशे नक्तमृज्रः।।९।।

By day he appears hari, (Lord Krishan) by night silvery white.

VIII_6^5

Oha, stadhasya titvishya abdya yate, some vatra yata indra sharmavaya rushashi ||5||

His might is manifest, for Indra folds and unfolds both heaven and earth as a skin. He has cloven with a powerful hundred-edged thunder bolt-the head of turbulent vritra ||1||

As daughter mushrooms grow the upper cap of each mushroom, as it were fold and unfold itself, appearing as a cloven - hoof, finally the cap attaining a red-orange colour.

$IX_{72}{}^{7}$ नाभा पृथिव्या धरुणो महो दिवोऽ्डपापूर्मी सिन्धुष्वन्तरुक्षितः।
इन्द्रस्य वज्रो वृषभो विभोवसुः सोमो हृदे पवते चारु
मन्सरः।।७।।

In the navel of the earth (is situated the soma) which is also the mainstay of the sky ||7||

In Hindu scriptures, it is depicted that Lord Krishan is always reclining with ease on the soft bed of several Seshnag (snake) while from his novel (umbilicus) arise a stalk of lotus (umbilica cord) This is a figurative way of explanation. Soma-plant is compared in the same metaphor.

$IX_{74}{}^{2}$ दिवोः स्कम्भो धरुणः स्वातत आपूर्णो अंशुः पर्येति
विश्वतः।
सेमे मही रोदसि यक्षदावृतान् मध्वो यंशुः पवत अन्द्रियाय।।६।।

Mainstay of the sky, well laid, the full amsu runs throughout everything ||2||

The mushroom generally arise from a humus-mould heap, the stalk originating as it were from novel of the earth, the cap opens and is like an inverted bowel (sky). This is a another way of suggesting the existence of a mushroom-plant.

$IX_{89}{}^{6}$ विष्टमभो दिवो धरुणः पृथिव्या विश्रवा उत क्षितयो हस्ते
अस्य।
उत्सो गृणते नियुत्चसन् मध्वो अंशुः पवत इन्द्रियाय।।६।।

Thou sittest in the vessels having been pressed for Indra, inebriating drink, which inebriates supreme mainstay of heaven (Soma), who gazes in the far distance ||6||

The mushroom, with its red, cap facing the sky, with the stalk acting as the mainstay between the earth and sky.

VIII_9^{19}

When the swollen stalks were milked like cows with (full) udder.

The stalks of the mushrooms are compared to the "udders of cow" since cell-sap or milk easily oozes out from them when they are crushed or squeezed.

IX_{107}^5 दुहान दधर्दिव्य मधुप्रियं प्रत्नं सधस्यमासदत् ।
आपृच्छ्यं धरुणं वज्यिर्बीति नृभि धृतो विचक्षणः ।। ५ ।।

Milking the clear sweetness from the divine udders.

Further the 'cap' of the mushroom is termed as 'Sira' or 'murdha' and is stated as follows in the stanza given below:

IX_{27}^3 एष नृभिर्बि नीयते दिवो मूर्धा वृषा सुतः ।
सोमो वनेषु विश्ववित ।। ३ ।।

The bull, heaven's head (murdhan) soma (is) pressed ||3||

IX_{68}^4 समातरस विचरन वाजयन्नपः प्रमोथिरः स्वधया पिन्वते पदम ।
अंशुर्यविन पिपिशे यतो नृभिः सजामिभिर्नसते रक्षते शिरः ।।४।।

While 'soma' enters into contact with the gingers of the priests, he protects his head (sirah) ||4||

IX_{93}^3 साक मुक्षो मर्जयन्त स्वसारो दशधीशस्य धीतयो धनुत्रीः ।
हरिः पर्यद्रवज्जाः सूर्यस्य द्रोणं ननक्षे अन्यो न वाजी ।।३।।

The udder o the cow is swollen, the wise juice is imbued with its streams. In the vessels, the cows mix with their milk with murdham ||3||

As 'cap' (head of the mushroom gets matured it attains a semi-circular shape not unlike the udder of cow', stalk, representing the nibbles, the cap is full of juice (not-unlike udders of cow)

I_{87}^{5}

We speak because of our descent from the ancient father, the tongue moves with 'eye'[5] of soma.

IX_{9}^{4} ससप्त धीतिभिर्हितो नद्यो अजिन्वदद्रुहः ।
या एकमक्षि वावृधुः ।।४ ।।

soma has encouraged the rivers, free of grief, which have strengthened his single eye ||4||

IX_{10}^{8} नाभ नाभि न आ ददे चक्षुश्चित सूर्ये सचा ।
कवेर पत्यमा दुहे ।।८।।

The eye is altogether with the sun.

IX_{10}^{9} अभि प्रिया दिवस्पदमध्वर्यु भिगुहा हितम् ।
सूरः पृयति चक्षसः ।।९।।

The sun (soma) looks with his eye towards dear places, with the highest place of heaven ||9||

IX_{97}^{46} एष्स्य ते पवत इन्द्र सोमश्चमूबु धरि उशते तदस्वान ।
स्वचर्क्ष रुथिरः सत्यशुष्मः कामो नयो देवतामसर्जि ।।४६ ।।

S (Soma) who has 'eye'..... the sun. The mushroom, with its 'cap' is regarded as a 'red eye' not unlike the sun.

X_{9}^{1} आपो हिष्टा मयोभुवस्ता न उर्जे दधातन ।
महे रवाय चक्षससे ।।१।।

ten slender young daughters seize him in the fray (soma), - the sister's on a decisive day.

The mushroom, (soma) is then taken by the head-priest or

priestess and with his or her long slender fingers of both hands (ten fingers) squeeze the plant, on a decisive day.

In Hindu - System of Medicine, extraction of drugs from plants are always done at certain 'Nakshatras' i.e. following certain position of sun, in the meridian. It is said that in particular position of the sun, in respect of Earth, active constituents within the plants vary and are at their optimum level, at certain times of a particular day.

IX_1^8 तमी हिन्वन्त्सग्रुणो धमन्ति बाकुरं हतिम्।
त्रिधातु वारणं मधु ।।८।।

The fingers push him (forward), thus to the place of pressing squeeze, shining leather bag-like stalk, this maead become possessed of three places (& becomes) the dispeller of enemies.

From the above stanzas it is explicit that when the mushroom are pressed, and completely extracted of sap, the plants shows a placid leather-like residue of the outer remains.

At times, the mushrooms are processed into wooden squeezers with iron grills, contraption not unlike wooden rollers used for crushing sugar-cane sticks for extraction of juice. This device has an outlet leading to a fleecy filter (wool), so that the juice as it flows gets clearly filtered.

This is clearly noted the stanzas recorded below:

IX_1^2 रक्षोहा विश्वचर्बणिरभि योनिम्योहतम्।
दुणा सधस्य मासदत् ।।२।।

The demon-killer, to whom all people belong, has seated himself on his seat on the wood towards his iron-hewn place of origin.

IX_3^9 एब प्रत्नेन जन्मना देवो देवेभ्यः सुतः।
हरि पवित्रे अर्षीति ।।९।।

This god, pressed for the gods, by the ancient the reddish yellows, runs into the strainer 9

IX_5^9 त्वष्टारमग्रजां गोपां पुरोयावानमा हुवे।
इन्दुरिन्दो वृषा हरिः पवमानः प्रजापति।।९।।

I invoke, Tvastr, the first-born, the protector of people, going at the head, the yellow-coloured, the flowing Indu (Soma) becomes Indra, the showerer, the protector of people. 9

IX_7^6 अव्यो वारे परि प्रियो हरिर्वनेषु सीदसि ।
रेभो वनुष्यते मती ।।६।।

The yellow-coloured (Soma), dearest, mixed in the waters, sits on the (seat) made of the sheep-hair, the one producing sound, is attended by praise ||6||

IX^7_7 स वायुमिन्द्रमश्विना साफ मदेन गच्छति ।
रणा यो अस्त्य धर्मभिः ।।७।।

O Soma, clothe thee with milk for the exhilaration of the god-being sent towards the sheep-hair and water ||7||

IX_1^6 पुनाति ते परिस्त्रुतं सोमं सूर्यस्य दुहिता ।
वारेण शश्वता तना ।।६।।

Soma, flows on with pleasant stream, a Bull is devoted o the God.

IX_{30}^4 प्रसोमो अतिधारवा पवमानो असिष्यदत् ।
अभि द्रोणान्या सदम् ।।४।।

The soma, the pavamana, has flown over with stream towards the wooden rollers to sit ||4||

IX_{15}^6 एब बसूनि पिन्दना परुषा यथिवो अति ।
अव शदेषु गच्छति ।।६।।

(Soma) having gone beyond the shining twing-knots sticking, goes down into the pitchers ||6||

From the fore-going stanzas, it is clear that the plant(s) was squeezed or twisted in knots between the wooden rollers, lined by iron plates so that the juice is fully expressed, it runs through wool filters before falling into pitchers (droneas).

IX_{32}^{4} अभे सोमावचाकशन् मृगो न तक्तो अर्षसि ।
सीदन्नृतस्य योनिमा ।।४ ।।

O Soma-illuminating both (Heaven & Earth) thou runnest like a doer urged on.... thou sitting on the place of *Rta*.

IX_{42}^{1} जनयन रोचना दिवो जनयन्नप्सु सूर्यम् ।
वसानो गा अपो हरिः ।।१ ।।

Creating the Heaven's light, generation the sun in the waters, the reddish-yellow-clothing himself in milk and waters________ ||1||

IX^{3}_{57} स सर्मृजान आयुभिरिभो राजेव सुव्रतः ।
श्येनो न वसु षीदति ।।३ ।।

He being cleaned by men, like the elephant-king possessing excellent wonderful activities, sits in the cups like a hawk ||3||

IX^{5}_{5} अदातैर्जिहते बृहद द्वारो देवी र्हिरण्ययीः ।
पवमानेन सुष्टुताः ।।५ ।।

Doors, the golden goddess, go-(open) wide up, with their extensions shining well-praised by pavamana (Soma) ||5||

IX_{8}^{6} पुनांनः कलेशेष्वा वस्त्रप्व्यरुषो हतिः ।
परिगव्यान्नव्यत ।।६ ।।

Being purified in the pitchers, the red-brown one has enveloped himself in garments of milk ||6||

From the above stanzas, it is clear that the reddish-brown

juice after being expelled by the wooden rollers, pass into the sieve of wool, and it collected in dronas or cups during this process, water and milk is continuously added.

Qualities

The merits of the expressed juice from soma-plant are quoted as follows:

VIII_8^4 आ नो यातं दिवस्वर्यान्तरि क्षादध प्रिया।
पुनः कव्वस्य वामिह सुषाव सोम्यं मधु।।४।।

Mitra, Varuna, I take soma, when sun is risen - it is medicine for sick ।।4।।

VIII_4^9 अश्वी रथी सुरुप इद् गोमा इदिन्द्र ते सखा।
श्वात्रभाजा वयसा सचते सदाचन्द्रो याति सभामुप।।९।।

Aśvins, for you with song of praise this hot oblation is effused. This your sweet Soma juice, you Lords of wealth, through which you think upon the foe.

IX_{25}^5 अरुषो जनयन गिरः सोम पवत अयुषक्।
इन्द्रं गच्छन् कवि क्रतुः।।५।।

The reddish (Soma), generating songs, flows on accompanied by vigour, (he) of wise, intelligence going to Indra ।।5।।

VIII^6_6 वि चिद् वृत्रस्य दोधातो वज्रेण शातपर्वणा।
शिरो बिभेद वृष्णिना ।।६।।

The soma juice increase vigour, intelligence, cure diseases and rejuvenates the human body, and naturally one begets healthy offsprings.

VIII_4^{10} ऋष्यो न तृष्यन्नपावमा गहि पिबा सोमं वर्शो अनु।
निमेघमानो मधवन् दिवेदिव ओष्टिं दधिघे सह।।१०।।

Like a thirsty stag, comes to drink Drink soma, as much as you wish. Pissing it out day by day. O, generous one- you have assumed a mighty force ||10||

IX_8^5 देवेभ्यस्त्वा मदायकं सृजातमतिमेष्यः ।
सं गोभ वसियामसि ।।५।।

Thee being sent forward beyond the sheep-hair (wool), for the exhilaration of gods-clothe over with milk ||5||

IX_{74}^4 आत्मन्वन्नभो दुष्यते घृतं पय ऋतस्य नाभिरमृत विजायते ।
समीचीनाः सुदानवः प्रीणन्ती तं नरो नितमवमेहन्ति
पेरवः ।।४।।

Further from the above stanzas it is clear that after drinking of the soma-juice decoction of milk, one gets frequent calls for urination (diuretic), more-so the individual gets exhilarant .

Habitat

Soma plant is found in moist situations and the verses below records the description:

IX_5^4 वर्हि प्राचीन मोजसा पवमानः स्तृणन् हरिः ।
देवेषु देवईयते ।।४।।

The thousand streamed (soma) (Pavamana) sits down amongst us on his mother lap in water and has spread in the ground ||4||

IX_1^5 त्वामच्छा चरामसि तदिदर्थं दिवेदिवे ।
इन्दो त्वे न आशसः ।।५।।

Pure soma, consecrate with thy streaming ambrosia, the yellow-golden hued Vanaspati with its thousand branches ||5||

The mushroom at its base gives several thousand gugal hyphae (Branches), which spread out in the moist substratum. The mushroom is orange-red in colour.

Search for Soma-plant

Aryans were known to have migrated to India, from various routes, some from Mediterranean regions, others from vast plains of Siberia, through the land routes via Turkey., Iran and Afghanistan into northern region of India, traversing the mountain passes of Khyber and Bolan, or they may have crossed the Himalayas at certain vintage points, now lost in oblivion. What plant they bring with them for rejuvenation from old-age and sickness has been described in Vedic texts.

Aryan civilisation*[6] in its peak of prosperity and development, indulged into this hallucinogenic drink obtained from Soma. The plant was known only to those who read the texts & the scriptures and these were only the priests or Brahmins.

Several centuries afterwards, barbarian tribes entered India and laid waster to all the remembrances of the Ancient Civilization.

It is wrong to assume that there was vacuum in Indian thought and knowledge. The Vedas have been rewritten, often newer ideas were interpolated to exploit the ignorant masses by the priests. Then came revival and systematic study of Plants, in modern era, and then only when the texts were pursued by botanists, did the identification of this plant became possible.

Hooker[7] mapped the Angiospermic Vegetation of India; Royle[8] recorded plants of the Himalayan Mountains, but they fully ignored the Mushrooms, even the encyclopedic work of Watt[9] did not take any cognizance of the fungal flora. So much so the later Ayurvedic Medical texts seem to have completely over-looked the original description of the plant.

Susruta Samhita[10] quotes description of soma-plant, which appears more that of substitutes used, than of the authentic plant in question. The details given by them are as follows:

"A soma-plant of what-ever varieties (there are 24 varieties), is furnished with 15 leaves which waxes and wanes with the phases of Moon.* Thus one leaf grows every day in the lighted

---

* Moon, in Sanskrit mean "Soma".

fortnight attaining the greatest number 15; in the night of full moon and then the leaves bare stem of creeper is left on the night of new Moon".

This description of the plant is an hypothetical version, by those who did not have the faintest idea of the plant in question but wanted to cover up their ignorance. The succeeding generation of priests took course, to regard cimbers (Valli) as their soma-plant. Of the substitute well recognised were. (1) *Periploca aphylla* DC. (2) *Ephedra vulgaris* Ṙich and (iii) *Sarcostemma brevistigma* W.A.

In later additions of stanzas of Rig-Veda we find still very interesting records:

$X_{85}3$ सोमं मन्यते पपिवान यत सापिषन्न्योबधिम् ।
सोमं त्रं ब्रम्हाणो विदुर्न तस्याश्रनाति कश्चन ।।३ ।।

One thinks one drink soma, because a plant is crushed;
the soma that the Brahmins know not, one drinks. ||3||

It indicates that priests knew less about the plant and offered substitutes instead.

Identification

The description as recorded in poetic metaphors, about the soma-plant in Rig Vedas tallies to a Mushroom called *Amanita*. Credit of identifying the plant goes to Dr. Wasson[14] an ethmo-mycologist of United States.

Soma-plant in Modern Terminology

Amanita muscaria 15a, 15b, It is a mushroom, commonly called Fly-agaric. It blooms generally in autumn, after rains, especially in pure and poplar woods of Siberia. The cap is orange-red in colour (cf. Plate...), sometimes at maturity caps are as large as 10 to 16 cm. in diameter. Some Siberian tribes eat the mushrooms to produce state of intoxication. The name fly-mushroom of fly-agaric has been given to it because it was once employed for preparing fly-poison, by boiling some slices of mushroom in milk.

Chemistry and Pharmacology

A powerful alkaloid muscarine has been recently from *Amanita muscaria* and its related species. The effects of the alkaloid are found to be similar to those of pilocarpine especially on the autonomic nervous system.

Muscarine is a quarternary ammonium base and related to chlorine. It shows senere toxic properties.

Recently psychotropic principles have been extracted and purified[16] Muscarin is a tetra-methylammonium derivative of a tetrahydrofuran.[17] The active compounds are muscazone[18] which has an oxazole structure; ibotenic acid,[19] a novel amino-acid containing the isoxazole ring and muscimol[20] which is derived from the previous compound by loss of carbon-dioxide. These substances are also found in other species of *Amanita* and *Inocybe* mushrooms. They produce marked effects on brain, causing mid-brain sedation and cortical excitation, resulting in a mild hypnotic state, accompanied by hallucinations and hyper-anesthesia.[21]

(1) Ibotenic acid.
(2) Muscimol.
(3) Muscazone.
(4) Muscarine.

Some compounds causing gastro-enteric disturbances needs further investigations.

Symptoms

On ingestion of a portion of mushroom[22], in about ten to fifteen minutes, the patient gets drowsy, with attack of gastro-enteristis, accompanied by emesis. At times, mild sedation follows within two hours or so, the patient wakes up with elation, hyperkinesis, starts speaking, or shouting finally showing signs of visual hallucinations. Sometimes the central excitement persists for a few hours, and in some it is much longer.[23]

On the other hand, Ibotenic acid, or pantherine have been noticed not to produce gastro-enteritis. Experiments on human beings[24] (using pure substances) showed that 20 mg. of ibotenic acid brings about facial flushing, lassitude and a severe occipital headache, lasting nearly for two weeks. A dose of 10 mg. muscimol produces dizziness, ataxia, euphoria, change in vision colour, and myoclonic twitching. Further increase in dosage upto 15 mg.

brings about in about thirty to forty minutes, dizziness, slight anorexia, visual echo pictures, auditory echo, and myoclonic cramps lasting for nearly four hours, *Treatment* : A simple gastric lavage, to control severe hallucinations, chlor-promazine may be employed.

Other species of the Mushroom

There are nearly twelve species of *Amanita*[24b] so far known, with a possibilities of others.

These are:

1. *Amanita pantherina* (Fr.) Secr.—Panther Amanita.
2. *Amanita flavivolva* Murr.
3. *Amanita cothuunata* Atk.—Booter Amanita
4. *Amanita phalloides* (Fr.) Secr. —Death cup.
5. *Amanita verna* (Fr.) Vitts. Bond —Spring Amanita
6. *Amanita virosa* Secr. The destroying Angel
7. *Amanita bisporigera* Atk.
8. *Amanita brunnescens* Atk.
9. *Amanita tenuifolia* Murr.
10. *Amanita verniformis* Murr.
11. *Amanita virosiformis* Murr.
12. *Amanita muscaria* (Fr.) Hook-Fly Agaric. *

In addition to hallucinogenic constituents present in these species, there are found amino-acids like noradrenaline, dopamine, and 3-methoxy-tyramine which also act as regulators of the central nervous system.

Amanita phalloides contains a toxic polypeptides[25] phalloidin[26] and amanitin[27,28] These are cyclic polypetides, containing in addition to common aminoacids, hydroxytryptophane, dihydroxy-leucine, hydroxyleucine and other amino-acids.

In Amanitin and Phalloidin one finds presence of an S-bridge, between a cysteine and a tryptophane residue.

The mode of action of these substances are yet to be elucidated and probably they interfere with some essential enzymatic cycle. Although these are toxic for man their LD in the mouse is rather high. Proteobytic enzymes have now[50] found use in modern therapy.[29]

---

* Toxicity of some of the above mentioned species needs further verification.

References

2. Tilak, B.G.: 1955. The Orion or researches into the Antiquity of Vedas. 4th Edition. Poona.
3. De Terra, H and Patterson, T.T. (1939): Studies on the Ice-Ages in India and associated Human cultures Carnegie Inst. Publ. 493. Washington.
4. Dey, N.L. (971): The geographical dictionary of Ancient and Mediaeval India. Oriental Book Reprint Corp. New Delhi.
5. Japanese God gave birth to sun-Goddess, while washing out his eyes. Ptah, proto-god of Egyptians fathered gods through his eyes, Hebrews say God, made light, then added God-was light and his symbol was the eye. Eye is an emblem of sun-God and gate-way of soul: Brit Med. J.1 : 170; (1971).

*6. Maya culture flourished in America, some 4,000 years (?) ago, they worshipped Mushroom, as their God. (cf.... Plate..) As recorded earlier, Asia, Siberia and America, were inter-connected by land-bridges. It is quite possible that this mushroom cult spread in the Siberia and then brought to India by early Aryans (!)

7. Hooker J.D. (1872-97): Flora of British India Vols. 1-7, London.
8. Royle J. Forbes: (1839): Illustrations of the Botany and other branches of Natural history of the Himalayan Mountains of the flora of Cashmere, London.
9. Watt G: (1889-99): Dictionary of the Economic Products of the India.
10. Susruta Samhita: (1939) Susrutacharya N.S. Press. Bombay.
11. Karnick, C.R. (1969): True identity of 'Soma-Plant' the famous Ayurvedic rejuvenating and longevity promoting Drug: Nag-Arjun 12: (11): 25-32.
12. Ali. U.S. and Narayanaswami V. (1970) Soma: Jour. Res. Ind. Med. 5: 106-113.
13. Srivastava.
14. Wasson, R.G: Soma-Divine mushroom of immortality Harcourt. Brace and World. New York.

15a. Atkinson, G.F. (1900-1969): Mushrooms-Edible Poisonous, etc. -thaca-Andrus and Chirch.

15b. Kriger, L.C.C. (9167) The Mushroom Hand-Book, Dover Publications Inc, New York.

16. Eugster, C.H. (1958) Helv. Chem. Acta. 41, 886 (1958).
17. Kogl, F; H.C. Cox, and Salemink, C.A.: (1957) Experientia 18, 137 (1957).
18. Fritz. H: AR. Gagneus; R. Zbinden: C.H. Eugster (1965) Tetrahedron Letters 7: 2075.
19. Eugster, C.H: G.F.R. Muller, and R. Good (1965) Tetrahedron Letters. 7, 1813.
20. Onda, M; H. Fukushima, and M. Akagawa: 91965) Chem. Pharm. Bull. (Tokyo) 12, 751.
21. Waser, P.G: In Ethno-pharmacologic search for psycho-active drugs 91967) U.S. public Health. Serv. Publ. N. 1965. Washington.
22. Lampe, K.F. and R. Fagerstrom (1968) Plant toxicity and dermatitis. The Wiolliams and Wilkims co. Baltimore.
23. Roch, M. and J.P. Mach (1960) Delire grave et prolonge cause par un empoisonnement par *Amanita Muscaria* (fause orange) Praxis. 49: 266.
24. Waser, P.G.: (967) The pharmacology of *Amanita muscaria* in Ethni-pharmacologic search for physcho-active drugs. Proc. symposium. San. Franceso. Calif. Jan 28-30. U.S. Dept. Heldth, Education and Welfare. U.S. Govt. Printing Office.

24b. Krieger, C.C.L. (1967): The mushroom hand-book Dover. Publ. inc. New York.
25. Wieland. Th: (1949) 564:152.
26. Wieland Th, and H.W. Schnabel: 1962) Ann. 657: 218
27. Wieland Th: Pure: (1964) Appl. Chem. 9: 145.
28. Wieland Th and U. Gebert: (1966) Amm 700: 157.
29. Tyler, V.E. Jr.: Recent studies on the chemical constituents of the Agarcicles. Beitrage zurbiochemic and physiologic von naturstoffen, Festschrift. Kurt. Mothes Zum. 65. Geburtstag. Gustav. Fisher. Verlang. Jena. (1964) 501.

III

CANNABIS

Cannabis is another well-known drug-plant mentioned in the Ancient Hindu Medical Classics, the Atharva Veda[1a] (1400 B.C.).

It has a mythological origin, and is said to have been brought from "Kailas", the highest peak of the Himalayas, by Lord Siva for his disciples, to attain mental bliss. More-over, it is said to one of the favourite drinks of Lord Indra. He sent it on the earth to banish fear, and encourage those who wished to attain `nirvana' or `mental bliss'.

The term 'Bhang' or 'gatra-bhanga'[1b] in Sanskrit, literally means, "body-disintegrator" since there is a belief that 'body' could be set free from mental plane, by the use of this drug so much so it disintegrates the normal human senses (Atharva Veda IX_{34}^{6})

India, a land famous for spiritual teaching and practice, is full of ascetics and religious mendicants. They use it with a belief that this drug may help them in concentration of mind and meditation.

Bhang is closely associated with many Hindu rituals namely the decoction of the leaves with milk is drunk on the 'Shiv-ratri' day. It is often distributed among guests as milk-shakes, on auspicious days of Durga puja festivals.

The use of Bhang, as an intoxicant has been going on for several centuries. It has been used to banish fear, deaden starvation pains, induce courage during fights with invaders, etc.

The term 'Bhang' has another meaning in Sanskrit. It is 'ananda' which denotes delightness; harshini i.e. wonderful or 'madini' sex intoxicator; ganjakini i.e. Vibrator etc., all referring in one way or the other to the qualities of the drug.

Plant

Cannabis sativa Linn (Family *Cannabaceae*) is an annual herb. (at times perennial), reaching an optimum height of 5 meters in wild state. It is erect, branched, and tap-rooted. *Stems* polygonal or rounded in cross-sections, ribbed or furrowed, hollow inside at maturity, scabrous, covered with resinous dots (glands), on young parts of the axis. *Leaves*: decussate, at base; alternate at upper ends; palmately compound 3 to 15, in some case 5 to 9, coarsely serrate, long lanceolate leaf-lets; the lower surfaces of which are pale-green, covered with yellowish-brown resinous glands (dots) and strigose hairs; the upper surfaces, dark-green, covered with stiff, bulbous conic trichomes.

Plants dioecious, dimorphic; *staminate plants*-tall slender with a few leaves in their terminal inflorescences; *carpellate plants*: stocky, with a dense crown of leaves associated with inflorescences.

Staminate inflorescences : in loose cymose panicles, originating from the axils of foliage leaves. Staminate flowers pedicellate small caducous. Tepals green quincuncial in buds, wide-spread at anthesis.

Carpellate inflorescences : In close axillary spikes in the main axis; leaves, petioles and bracts of carpellate inflorescence, densely covered with resinous capitate and sessile glandular haurs. Carpellate flowers sessile ensheated by a glandular beaked perigynal bracteole and subtended by a bract.

Perianth papery closely appressed to ovary. Fruit: Ovoid compressed achne with persistent perianth mottled with brown spots. Pericarp: 5 layered inner palisade layer thick. Seed one, ovoid, perisperm one-called layer, layer thick. Seed one, ovoid, perisperm one-called layer, endosperm fleshy, with a chalazal haustorium embryo curved C-shaped, flexed in the region of the epicotyl with radicle and octyledon tips pointing towards the micropylar end of the seed; Chromosomes number, 2n = 18 + XX or XY.

The plant is distributed throughout the world and is indigenous to Central Asia 31, 35. *Cannabis* has a long history of cultivation for its hemp fibres[3,4,5].

Botanically[6] speaking, a single species has been recognised i.e. *C. sativa* Linn. but another species has been found in United

States, namely C. *ruderalis*[2] Jan. There is still much void in the knowledge about the various races of *Cannabis* occurring in different parts of the world.

The plant is influenced much by variations in climate[7] temperature[8] soil time of harvest, conditions of height etc.[9]

The plant contain resin in its resin-glands which are spread on all the parts, especially, the flowering axes, and juvenile leaves of male and female plants[10,11].

Chemistry

Neumeyer and Shagorory[12] has recently reviewed theoretically the active principles present within the plant. These are cannabinoids, waxes, starches, terpenses, oil and traces of unidentified substances. Of the important Cannabinoids are the (-)-Δ^9*Pharmacology* : transtetrahydrocannabinol (Δ^9—THC)[13]; (-)-Δ—transtetrahydrocannabinol (Δ^8—THC)[14] and Δ^9—transtetrahydrocannabinolic acid (THC-acid), cannabinol (CBN) and cannabidiol (CBD). The former two are psycho-active if used orally or smoked. THC-acid becomes activated to Δ^9 or Δ^8 when smoked[13]. CBN and CBD are present in large amounts, exact nature of action is still unknown.

Δ^8 —THC is more active than Δ^9 —THC[14] Δ^9 —THC is principally, the one which brings about most of the effects of *Cannabis*. It is the pharmacological active compound. Mechoulam[13] isolated nearly thirty other cannabinodis and much about their biological activity is still to be known. *Cannabis* also contains alkaloids[15] which show atropine-like, and trigonelline like activity.

Smoking causes Δ^9 —THC and Δ^8 —THC. to volatilizes and gets into the human lungs.[16] They are also absorbed by gastro-intestinal tracts, while in experimental animals, it was found that Δ^9 —THC and Δ^8 THC generally adhere to serum protein. Strangely enough even a small quantity enters the brain, while in liver, they get metabolized. These metabolites[17] generally get exerted in the bile. These get re-absorbed in gastro-intestinal tract, recording entero-hepatic circulation.

The metabolites[17] of Δ^9 —THC and Δ^8 —THC in liver turn into 11-hydroxyl derivates i.e. (11-OH-Δ —THC and 11-OH-Δ^8 THC). Additional hydroxylations occurs on the rings. The 11-hydroxyl derivatives of Δ^9 —THC and Δ^8 —THC are the only pharmacological active constituents.[18] The metabolites are found to remain within the bodies of experimental animals for a considerable length of time.

Klausner and Doingell[19] noticed that Δ^8 —THC and Δ^9 —THC disappear from blood readily with practically no trace after fifteen minutes, in intravenous injections to the experimental animals.

A comparison of synthetic tetrahydro-cannabinols namely (1) (±) $\Delta^{6a,10a}$ THC; (2) (±) $\Delta^{6a\text{-}5\text{-}n}$ hexyltetrahydrocannabinol (synthexyl or parahexyl) and (3) (±) (DHMP), showed that the former one, of the synthetic tetrahydrocannabinol recorded only 1/14 of the biological activity of the natural Δ^9. THC (loewe[20]) while the second one, synhexyl possess, cannabis-like activity and act as anti-depressant[21]. The last one, DHMP. was found to the quite potent drug, in doses of 1 to 2 mg. orally in man. It reproduced, cannabis-like effects, marked sedation and extreme postural hypotension.

The contents of cannabinoids in any seizure materials, can be easily estimated by gasliquid chromatography.[22,23,24,25,26,27]

Δ^9 THC contents of Cannabis preparations are influenced by many factors, viz. growth, age, climate, soil, etc.

Epidemiology

A recent symposium[28] of the Indian Council of Medical Research on the long term effects of *Cannabis* use in India, brought the following facts to light.

1. Manner of intake, different preparations, frequency, dosage, etc.[29]

The usual mode of consummation of *Cannabis* in India is either by smoking, direct ingestion of grounded leaves in form of pills, or by drink, as milk-shakes. It is unique, that 'Bhang' is either taken as beverage or smoked. Various confections contain mixtures of leaves in various proportions. The following types have been recognised.

I *Bhang*:[30,31,32].

(i) *Pill*-Bhang (*Cannabis*) is grounded or pounded to form a "bolus", from fresh leaves of female plants and flowers, this is consumed directly by the users.

(ii) *Drink*-Fresh leaves of *Cannabis* are pounded together with several ingredients like black-pepper, rose petals, poppy seeds, melon seeds, cucumber seeds, almonds, cardamon, cloves, cinnamon bark pieces, senna leaves, and saffron. The powdered mass is then mixed in milk and consumed as milk-shakes.

The quantity of ingredients vary according to individual needs. Generally each individual takes one glass-ful of this "Bhang-shake".

In Punjab and U.P. this milk decoction is known as 'hand', 'thandai', and 'sawi', while in Bengal it is known as 'sidhi', in Maharashtra and Madhya Pradesh as 'ghota' or bhang, while in Rajasthan it goes by the name of 'dudhi" and in South India (Kerala and Tamil Nadu) as "Raruras" or 'Ram-Rasain'.

(iii) *Confections* : Special preparations of *Cannabis* sold in Indian bazars are:

(I) *Majum*: In this preparation, leaves of *Cannabis* are fried or boiled in water, and when a green paste is obtained, it is mixed with condensed milk, khoua or mawa and finished product is sold as "Barfi".

(II) *Halwa* : This is another kind of preparation made by boiling *Cannabis* leaves in sugar syrup, wheat flour is added and a sort of pudding is prepared.

(III) *Curry* : In villages of Tamil Nadu and Kerala, leaves of *Cannabis* are used in curries of various kinds, viz. in 'Churnam', pillai legiyam', 'Purnadhi legiyam', 'majiyam and "Purnadhi", etc. and generally taken with rice.

(IV) *Chewing*: Juvenile fresh leaves of *Cannabis* are chewed by Purbhayas, and milk, vendors of Maharashtra, etc. They do so to get relief from strenuous night-duties.

II *Ganja*[33]

It is a more potent drug than Bhang, and is a mixture of dried flowering and fruiting tops of female plants covered with resinous exudes from glandular hairs. Three varieties are produced in India and these are (i) *flat* (ii) *round* and (iii) *choora*. *Flat ganja* is prepared by spreading out dried plants with resin on floor and pressing them into sheets.

On pounding, the material becomes glutinous with powdered fragments of leaves stems flowers and fruits, covered with resin. It is then made into circular cakes or disks called

'Chakk', height of which sometime reaches to one metre. It is generally kept in open. At times due to low quality of material, they are then prepared into sausage shaped masses by hand or even rounded into small balls, or pressed into flat discs. This variety is then known as *flat* ganja. At times the residue of round ganja is boiled in water ending up in homogeneous granules. These are marketed as 'Choora ganja'.

III *Charas*

It is much superior variety in potency than the former two products and mostly contain resinous material collected from the glandular leaves and flowering tops of female plants. The high quality of charas or hashish* comes from Central Asia and Chinese Trukistan. This is usually smuggled in India and into the various countries of the world.

Techniques Followed in India

(i) *Smoking*: Ganja and Charas are smoked. Smoking is done in small red-clay pipes called "Chillum". It is a small red-clay pipe shaped more or less like a funnel but with wider base and narrower top. At lower end of this pipe usually they attach a piece of wet tobacco is introduced over which is piece of charcoal or smouldering cow-dung cake is placed, from the moistened cloth end of chillum held in between the palms, smoke is drawn into the mouth, through wet piece of cloth. This smoke is usually retained in the buccal cavity and released through the nostrils.

Not infrequent, ganja and charas is smoked in "hookah" a device exactly like `Chillum' but attached to a bowel containing water. The smoke is drawn in through water.

The crude-forms are less potent and are usually smoked in pipes or in cigarettes.

The most important aspect is the pattern of use. It is often admixtured with other drugs namely scopolamine, atropine and other belladonna with the stuff to make the effects stronger.

---

* *Cannabis sativa* Linn is known as 'Bhang' or *Ganja* (in India) *Kif* (in Algeria, and Morroco), Takrousi (in Tunis), Kabak, Asarath, Nasha (in Trukey), Hashish el Keif (in Suria and Lebanon), Djamba, Liamba, Riamba (in Central Africa and Brazil), Dagga (in South Africa), Marihuana (in North America), Suruma (in Mozambique), Rongony (in Madagascar) and Maconha (in Brazil).

Srivastava[35] carried out a survey of semi-urban communities in Varanasi on 728 adults and found that as much as 2.75 percent of adult population were regular users, whereas 4.12 per cent used ganja and charas in combination. 'Fakirs and Sadhus' are found at practically all religious places especially on the banks of rivers, these individual indulge in smoking ganja.

Reasons for use of Cannabis

General causes[35-41] attributed are a close association with habitual users, curiosity of effects, desire for relaxation, relief from tensions and alleviation of hunger.

The use of *Cannabis* in religious ceremonies are common in various cultural groups of Central and South Africa[42], Brazil[43], Jamaica[44], Mexico[45], etc.

In a recent study of Varanasi[35] community at Benaras, *cannabis* addition appeared to occur in two distinct groups of individuals. First group consisted of adults and middle-aged villagers where *Cannabis* plant was freely available. The second group comprised of adolescents and teen-agers in higher socio-economic strata from high-schools and colleges often associated with delinquency traits, weak parent-child relationship, unsatisfactory scholaristic career, homo-sexual activity or other promiscuous sex activities, addiction to other drugs like barbiturates, amphetamines and alcohol, was common within the group.

Singh[46] in his recent survey of Chandigarh population observed that 58.33 percent took up drug for curiosity, 55 percent for sake of moving along with newer gentlemen, 52 percent for relief of tensions, 41 percent for enjoyment, 33 percent for sex, 26 percent for getting work energy and 28 percent, because they liked its intoxication.

Dosage and Frequency

Much of the intoxicating effects of *Cannabis* depends upon the potency of the preparations used. It is extremely difficult to determine exactly the effect of a particular dose, much also depends on age, health and various other conditions of the user. Generally the effect of oval consumption is slow, milder, and longer in duration. The lethal dose of *Cannabis* has yet to be established in human beings. Fatalities due to drug have never been reported. The active principle tetra-hydrocanabinols (THC) is insoluble in water and the drug so far never has been used by injection.

Clinical studies[47] have shown that Δ^9 —THC is best absorbed by inhalation and get rapidly distributed in various tissues. The radio-activity of the material has a plasma half-life of 56 hours. Metabolism is by hydro-xylation and many polar metabolities are fired. 20 to 30 percent of the metabolities are excreted by kidneys and the remainder lost in faces. Small dosage bring about tachycardia which can be blocked by beta-adrenergic blocking drugs. Larger doses produces mental confusion, and depersonalisation.

Chronic use produces cerebral atrophy as diagnosed by pneumoencephalography. In some cases it revealed that there was a minor lapses in memory with no permanent disorder[49].

A chillam contains 1 to 2 gm of Ganja which is equivalent to 30 to 60 mg of Δ^9 THC.

Dube[77], found that out of 566 admitted cases for psychosis in Mental Hospital at Agra, there were 134 users of *Cannabis* in which 11 percent were using it daily, while 34 percent quite often. He estimated that more than 24 gm. was consumed by a group at one sitting using two 'chilams'. On an average two to four g, was consumer per day by an individual.

Socio-cultural Factors

It appears from various studies made in India and elsewhere, that rapid socio-cultural change, involving industrialisation, urbanization, social conflicts, disregard of human values, regarding religion, moral ethics, indiscipline patterns, growth of city slums, and various degrees of social alienation are probable causes of the use of this drug[50,51,53].

Effect on Man

Δ^9 THC accounts for the major part of the pharmacological activity of Cannabis preparations. The percentage of Δ^9 THC, in *Cannabis* preparations varies Markedly. The potency of various preparations varies directly with their Δ^9 THC concentration.

Manno et al[53] found that the techniques used so far, for smoking, accelerates as much as 50 percent of Δ^9 THC in *Cannabis* to go in smoke, while the remaining 50 percent is converted either to CBN or CBD or both. Only 50 percent of a Marijuana cigarette smoke is absorbed by the lungs and constitutes the dosages actually delivered to the smoker.

Immediate Effects

Symptoms after taking Δ^9 THC or *Cannabis* preparations depends on the dose[54] as well as on mental condition and health of the user.

Researchers[55,56,57,58,59] have found in their experiments that a dose of 50 ug/kg by smoking or 120 ug/kg orally, caused mild euphorbia. Dose of 100ug/kg smoking or 240 ug/kg oral brought about perceptual and sensory changes. Dose of 200-250 ug/kg smoking or 300-480 ug/kg oral a marked distortion of sensory perception, depersonalization, derealization, optical and auditory hallucinations. If dose is increased between 30 and 70 mg (400 and 1000 ug/kg), with a median dose of 50 mg. (700 ug/kg)-the characteristic syndrome was euphoria, psychic changes generally followed by sedation and sleep.

Other signs in experimented individuals are conjunctivae, a decreased in muscular strength, slight increase in pulse rate, resting systolic and diastolic blood pressure, respiration rate, body temperature, pupil size remaining un-affected.

Cannabis users report auditory sensitivity and enhanced appreciation of music.[59]

Some users develop a subjective sense of enhanced touch, taste and smell[60] but measurements of threshold for touch, vibration, two pound discrimination, olfactory acuity, and visual brightness have shown no change[61]

Psychotoxic Reactions

High dosage brings about acute intoxication, setting in paranoid ideas, illusions, hallucinations, delusions, confusions, restlessness and excitement[62].

Recently Thacore[63] found in Lucknow cases of paranoid psychosis resulted from chronic "bhang" (*Cannabis*) use, resembling paranoid schizophrenia. The clinical picture was characterised by a hostile perception of the environment, fearfulness with delusions of persecution, auditory and visual hallucinations, occurring in a state of clear consciousness with no memory disturbance.

After-effects

Physical disorders

It has been noticed that smoking of 'Ganja' and 'Charas' over long periods of time, generally leads to various respiratory diseases, namely chronic bronchitis. Since *Cannabis* is used in several combinations, especially with tobacco, much less is known about the etiology of such conditions.

Studies by Sterne and Ducastaling[64] in Morocco, among the Moors who are heavy users of "Kif" (*Cannabis*), showed that the users suffered for arterists.

Madan[65] with his experiments on rats, found that *Cannabis* prolongs sleep and immobility with hexo-barhital and pento-barbital combinations. This he says is due to interference with microsomal degradation of barbiturates. Further, he observed that *Cannabis* lengthens hypnosis due to ethanol, augments amphetamine-induced arousal, hyperactivity, and potentiates the effects of caffeine. Further, he noticed that amphetamine synergizens the ataxia induced by *Cannabis* while cocaine antagonises the sedation caused by it., morphine enhances its CNS-depressant, and analgesic actions. Another reaction observed was that use of muricidal behaviour inhibited by atropine, haloperidol and diazepam.

Psychoses

Various psychiatric conditions appear with the use of *Cannabis*, covering a wide range of disorders and situations.[66]

Acute psychotoxic reactions occur with heavy intake of *Cannabis* lasting for 1 to 6 weeks only. Keeler and co-workers[67] found that in several cases, spontaneous recurrence of unusual somatic and visual sensations, were experienced after heavy intake of *Cannabis*.

Lysergide (LSD) user report occurrence of 'flash-back phenomena' some cases of *Cannabis* addicts, also record precipitation of flash-back phenomena in person who have taken LSD.[69] Constant users of *Cannabis*, for several years, show measurable deflicts in a number of psychomotor and cognitive functions.

Cannabis use in Teenagers

A study[70] on medical students, at Agra Mental Hospital showed that Cannabis use is most popular among younger students. This trend of indulgence arise in big cities, like Delhi, Calcutta, Bombay, etc., A study of 566 male admitted during one year at Mental hospital showed that 319 admission revealed the same trend.

This fact reveals that users are prone for experimentation of all kinds of chemical comforters, trying to ward off excessive strain and stresses of new technological society development, despair, conflicts, demandingness and social confrontations, etc.

Birdwood[71] states that teenagers who rely on drugs are more or less consciously detaching themselves from the society with which they are out of apathy. Some of these youngsters cannot cope, others fail to find a niche in it, still others gape at society with disenchanted looks, others simply wish to ignore it.

In fact, with ever-increasing unemployment, uncertainties of future, distorted social values, adolescence, behavioural patterns, go a long way in inculcating youngsters towards drug addiction.

Tolerance

It is an adaptive state characterised by diminished response to the same quantity of a drug.[72]

Experiments on animals have shown that a high degree of tolerance is developed to Δ^9 THC in pigeons[73], mice, rats and dogs[74]. Smokers of charas and ganja, who consume daily onan average of 720 mg. of Δ^9 THC develops a certain degree of tolerance.

Reference

1a. Whitney, I (1908) English translation of Atharva Veda. Harvard Oriental Series Vol. 7 & 8.

1b. Karnick C.R. (969) Genus Cannabis (Bhang, Ganja and Charas) the famous narcotic from India, with potentials for newer drugs. (A review): (unpublished).

2. Miller, N.G. (1970): The genera of the Cannabaceae in South-Eastern United States, Jour. Arnold, Arbor-51 (2): 185.

3. Indian Hemp Drug Commission (1894): Indian Hemp Drug Commission Report 1893-1894. Simla (1894).

4. Wealth of India (1948): CSIR publication, New Delhi Vol. C.

5. Bouquet, J. (1950): Cannabis: Bull Narcot. 2(4): 14-30.

6. Joyce, CR. B and S.H. Curry (1970): The Botany and Chemistry of Cannabis London.

7. Harata, K. (1928): Sex determination in hemp. Jour. Genet, 19: 65-79.

8. Kohler, D (1958): Die Entwicklung von Cannabis sativa unter dem Einfluss verschiedener Tageslagen Physiol Pl 11: 249-259.

9. Hayward, H.E. (938): The structure of Economic Plants, New York.

10. Valle, J.R., Lapa, A.J. and Barros, G.G. (1968): Pharmacological activity of Cannabis according to the sex of the plant J. Pharm. Pharmacol. 20: 798-799.

11. Fetterman, P., Keith, E.E. Waller, C.: Guerrero, O; Doorenbos, J and M. Quimbry (1970): A preliminary observation on the chemical definition of phenotype and variations in the content, versus age, sex and plant part J. Pharm. Sci.

12. Neumeyer, J.L. and Shagorory R.A. (1971): Chemistry and Pharmacology of Marijuana, J. Pharm, Sci. *60*, 1433.

13. Mechoulam, R (1970): Marihuana chemistry, *Science*: 168: 11591-1166.

14. Gill, E.W., Paton, W.D.H. and R.G. Pertwee (1970): Preliminary experiments on the chemistry and pharmacology of Cannabis: Nature (Lond) *228*: 134-136.

15. Lerner, M and J.T. Zeffert: 1968): Determination of tetrahydrocannabinol isomers in marihuana and hashish. Bull. Narcot. 20(2): 53-54.

16. Manno. J.E.; Kiplinger, G.F., Haine, S.E. Bennett. I.F. and R.B. Forney: Comparative effects of smoking marihuana or placebo on human motro and mental performance. *Clin. Pharmacol Ther. 11*: 808-815 (1970).

17. Ben-zvi, L; Mechoulam, R and S. Burstein; Identification through synthesis of an activeD^6-tetra-hydrocannabinol metabolite-J. Amer. Chem. Sec. 92: 3465-3469 (1970).

18. World Health Organization Technical Report Series 478 (1971).

19. Klausner, H.A. and Dingell, J.V: Studies on the metabolism and distribution of D^9 -tetrahydrocannabinol. Pharmacologist 12; 259 (1970).

20. Loewe, S : *Cannabis*—Workstoffe and pharmakologieder cannabinole, *Naunyn*—Schmiedebergs. *Arch. Exp. Path.* Pharmak: 211: 175-189 (1950).

21. Parker, C.S. a nd Wrigley, F: Synthetic Cannabis prep.

22. Adam R: Marihuana, Bull, N.Y. Acad. Med. *18*: 705-730 91942).

23. Todd, A.R. Chemistry of the hemp drugs-nature (Lond) 146: 829-830 (1940).

24. De Zeuw, R.A. Th. M. Malingre and F.W.H.M., Merkus: D^1 -Tetra-hydrocannabinolic acid an important component in the evaluation of Cannabis products, J. Pharm. Pharmac. 24: 1-6 (1972).

25. Mechoulam, R, and Y, Shivo: Hashish I: The structure of cannabidol-Tetrahedron *19*: 2073-2078 (1963).
26. Lerner P: Precise determination of tetrahydro Cannabinol in Marihuana and hashish. Bull. Narcot 21(3): 39-42 (1969).
27. Lerner, M: Zeffert, J.T: Determination of tetrahydrocannaninol isomers in marihuana and hashish. Bull. Narcot 20(2): 53-54 (1968).
28. Abstracts: ICMR -Seminar on long term effects of Cannabis use in India, Dec. 6,7,8 New Delhi (1972).
29. Dube, K.C: Epidemiolgical studies of cannabis users in India: Manner of intake, different preparations, etc., ICMR. Symposium Abstract. P. 13. (1972).
30. Chopra I.C. and Chopra, R.N.: The use of the cannabis drugs in India. Bull. Narcot. 9(1): 4-29 (1957).
31. Chopra, G.S: Man and Marihuana. Int. J. Addict. 4: 215-247 (1969).
32. Boquet, J: Cannabis. Bull-Narcot 3(1):
33. Chopra R.N. and I.C. Chopra: Drug-addiction. CSIR New Delhi (1965).
34. Boquet, J: Cannabis Bull, Narcot. 3 (1) : 22-45(1951).
35. Srivastava O.N.: Extent of Cannabis use in India ICMR Symposium, Dec. 1972.
36. Tart, C.T: Marhuana intoxication, common experiences: Nature (long): 226: 701-4 (1970).
37. Becker, H.S: Becoming a marihuana user. Amer. J. Social 59: 235-242 (1953).
38. Soueif, M.I: Hashish consumption in Egypt with special reference to psycosocial aspects. *Bull Narcot* 19(2): 1-12 91967).
39. Indian Hemp Drugs Commission Report. Simla (1894)
40. Chopra, R.N. and Chopra, G.S: The present position of hempdrug addiction in India. Indian J. med. Res. *31*: 1-19 (1939).
41. McGlothlin, W.H. and West; L.J: The marihuana problem and overview. Amer. J. Psychiat. 125: 370-378 (1968).
42. Chopra, G.S.: Man and Marihuana. Int. J. addict. 4: 215-247 (1969).
43. Batista, E : Subsidios para O estudio medico social da maconha. Rev. bras. Med. 16: 648 (1959).
44. Blum, R.H. and Associates: Drugs I. Society and Drugs. San fracises. Jossey Baass. (1969).
45. Livet, L: Les fumeurs de marijuana. ann. med-psychol. 10me, series 12: 257-267 (1920).
46. Sarbit Singh: Motivation and attitude toward drug use in chronic Cannabis users. ICMR Seminar 1972.
47. Seth U.K.: Clinical pharmacological aspects of *Cannabis* ICMR Seminar. New Delhi: 1972.
48. Dube, K.C.: Manner of intake, different preparations, frequency, dosage, etc. ICMR. Seminar, New Delhi (1972) (Dec 6-8).
49. Agarwal, A.K.: Physical and cognitive effect of chronic bhang intake ICMR Seminar, New Delhi (1972).
50. Blum, R.H. and Associates: Drugs I + II-Society and Drugs, San-Francisco. Jossey Bass (1969 a,b).
51. Popham, R.E.: A.R.F. research on drugs, other than alcohol. Toronto. Addiction Research foundation (1970).
52. WHO: report of WHO scientific Group. Technical Report series. Geneva p. 478 (1971).
53. Manno, J.E., Kiplinger, G.F., Haine, S.E., Bennett, J.F. and Forney, R.B.:

Comparative effects of smoking Marihuana or placebo on human motor and mental performance Clin. pharmacol. Ther. 11: 808-15(1970).

54. Hollister, L.E.: Richards, R.K. and Gillespie, B.A.: Comparison of tetrahydrocannabinol and synhexyl in man, Clin. Pharmacol. Ther 9: 783-791 91968).

55. Clark, L.D., Hughes, R and Nakashima, E.N. Behavioural effects of Marihuana experimental studies: Radh. gen. Psychiat. 23: 193-98 (1970).

56. Isbell, H., Gorodetsky, C.W: Jasmski, D. Clausen U; V. Spulak, F and Korte, F: Effects of (—)D^9 transterahydrocannabinol in Man. Psychopharmacologia (Bel.) 11: 184-188) (1967).

57. Lindemann, E: The nourophysiological effects of intoxicating drugs. Amer. J. Psychiat. 90: 1007-1037 91933-34).

58. Well. A.T. Zingerg, N.E. and Nelsen, J.M. Clinical and psychological effects of Marihuana in Man. Science 162: 1234-1242 (1968).

59. Walton, R.P.: Marihuana. America's New-drug problem. Philadelphia, Lippineott (1938).

60. Tart, C.T. Marihuana intoxication, common experiences Nature (Lond) 226: 701-704 (1970).

61. Caldwell, D.F.: Myers, S.A., Domino, E.F. and Murraim, P.C: Auditory and Visual threshold effects of Marihuana in Man, Perception skills. 29: 755-759 (1969).

62. Baker, A.A: and Lucas, E.G.: Some hospital admissions associated with Cannabis. Lancet: 1: 148 (1969).

63. Thacore, V.R: Paranoid psychosis following prolonged abuse of Cannabis ICMR Seminar New Delhi (72).

64. Sterne, J and Ducastang C: Lessarterites due Cannabis indica. Arch Mal. Cauer. 53: 143-147 (1960).

65. Madan, B.R: Inter-action of Cannabis with other psychotropic drugs, ICMR Seminar New Delhi (1972).

66. Defer, B and Diehl M.L: Les psychoses cannabigues aigues (a propos de 560 observations) Ann. med. psychol. 126 (2): 260-266 (1968).

67. Keeler, M.H., Reifler, C.B. and M.B. Liptzin: Spontaneous recurrence of marihuana effect. Amer J. Psychiat *125*, 384-386 (1968)

68. Frosch, W.A, Robbins, E & M. Stern: Untoward reactions to lysergic acid diethylamide (LSD) resulting in hospitalization. *New* Engl. J. Med. 273: 1235-1239 (1965).

69. Weil, A.T: Adverse reactions to Marihuana New Dengl. J. Med. 282: 977-1000 (1970).

70. Aditya Kumar: Cannabis use in younger persons present day problems a research issues. ICMR Seminar New Delhi-1972.

71. Birdwood, G. E.B.: Present-day problems and Remedies p. 385 (1970)

72. Eddy, N. Halbach, H, Isbell, H and M. Seevers: Drug dependence, its significance and characteristic Bull Wld Hlth. Org. *32* : 721-733 (1965).

73. Macmillan, D, H; Harris, L.S., Frankenheim, J.M. and Kennedy, J.S: 1-D^9 tetrahydrocannabinol in pigeons, tolerance to the behavioural effects. Science 169: 501-503 (1970).

74. Dewey, W.L. Harris, L.S., Howes, J.F. and Kennedy J.S.: Pharmacological effects of some active constituents of Marihuana. Pharamacologist *11*; 278 (1969).

IV

GENUS CANNABIS LINN

Cannabis Linn. is a monotypoc genus and it exhibits several growth forms and varieties.

In India, *Cannabis indica* Lamb. (Syn. *Cannabis Sativa* Linn.) is quite well known as a drug plant. It is a Vedic plant used in Indian system of Medicine and mentioned in Ancient Hindu Medical Classics.

The narcotic use was long known to Aryans, who migrated into India thousands of years ago. Its use spread to Africa, Southern and Northern America, Canada, reached Asia Minor, and ingressed into areas of Soviet Republic.

Drug addiction and abuse has in recent years reached such magnitude and proportions in various parts of the world, that the authors thought it would be worth to collect all information from Ancient Hindu literature regarding this, which speaks so much about it and to bring together all the modern facets of knowledge which lie scattered in different disciplines. This drug addiction seems to smother the very foundations of younger intelligentsia, who have taken freedom with this drug plant.

Furthermore, it would be of great interest to those who seek to tap newer potentialities and also to those who are mentally sick and seek relief from pains.

With this object in view, the present review tries to bring home all the comprehensive details about this genus.

Older Records

1. Ancient Hindu Classics

'Bhang' (*Cannabis*) is a drug has been mentioned in the, Ancient Hindu Medical Classic, the Atharva Veda, as early as 1400 B.C.

Sushruta Samhita[300] (1000 B.C.) records the use of plant as a drug for the accumulation of phlegm in the larynx.

Furthermore, it has a mythological origin and is said to have been brought from 'Kailas', the highest peak of the Himalayas by Lord Siva (a deity known among Hindus to bring about mental peace and salvation) for his disciples, to attain mental bliss. Moreover, it is said to be the favourite drink of 'Lord Indra', and he too sent it on to the earth to banish fear and encourage those who wish to attain 'nirvana'.

The term 'Bhang' or 'gatra-bhanga' in sanskrit literally means "body disintegrator", since it was a belief that 'body' or 'soma' could be set free from mind, by the use of this drug. Nevertheless, it was clearly indicated that it is the disintegrator of normal human senses. (Atharva Ved. IX : 34. 35).

India is a land of spiritualism, ascetic and religious mendicants who use it with a belief that this drug will help them in concentration of mind and meditation. Bhang' is associated with many rituals, namely it is drunk on the 'Shiv-ratri' day. In eastern Bengal, Bhang-sherbat is offered to guests on ending of Durga Puja festivals.

Ganja, another form of Cannabis drug, is used as offerings in Tarkeshwar temple on Shiv-ratri day and on festivals of Trinath Puja. It is drunk during Holi and Depavali festivals. Sikhs and Rajputs use it freely as offerings to devotees visiting their religious places and shrines.

Bhang has been used to induce a state of intoxication, to excite emotion, to encourage sense of bravado, during Rajput skirmishes and battles. These warriors, during their forced encounters with raiding Muslim hordes from North in last century, used bhang to banish fear and induce courage and deaden pain during fights.

Furthermore, intoxicating qualities of this drug are revealed by usage of certain Sanskrit terms, namely 'ananda' (means delightness); harshini (wonderful); 'madini' (sex intoxicator); ganja or 'ganjakini' (vibrator).

Among other oriental writings, Chinese were also known to us this drug plant even before 500 B.C.

2. Ancient European Classics

Scythians[238] appear to be well acquainted with this narcotic drug plant. As early as 2500 years. King Herodot (5th B.C.)

reports the use of vapours of 'Kavva Bis' for intoxication by Scythians, on the battle shores of Caspian Sea. Queen Helen has been forced to administer this drug to king Telmachus on the advice of king Homer. Female populace of Thebes used this drug to dissipate anger and melancholy of their ever angry spouses.

The consumption of *Cannabis* appears to have spread in Europe during second half of the last century, so much so, Baudelaire[40] describes his reminiscences with Bhang, in his famous book 'Les Paradis artificiels' and records the presence of the "Club des Hachichins" in Paris, where 'elite' for France use together.

Furthermore, during Napoleon's expedition to Egypt, qualities[322] of this drug were brought to his notice for giving patronage.

Watt[322] traces the history and details of the usage of this drug in India, later this is followed by the report of the first enquiry commission, based on scientific lines. This report[267] dealt with the prevalence addiction in India during 1893-94, with simultaneous experimentations carried out by O'Shanghnessy[252] in the usefulness and qualities of this drug and thus bringing it in use in Western Medicine.

Stuart[299] prepared a 'resume' on 'Ganja' with special reference to the effect of narcotic principle, tetrahydrocannabinol on man and test-animals, inasmuch, he has drawn attention to the anti-bacterial, analgesic anticonvulsive and local anesthetic effects of ganja extracts.

Chopra and Chopra[87] brought out a small memoir on drug addiction in India giving account of different drugs in which the study of *Cannabis* is included.

Mikuriya[238] published a very thought-provoking article on Marijuana. He states that medicine in the western world has forgotten almost all it once knew about therapeutic properties of *Cannabis*.

Origin and Distribution

De Candolle[75] suggested that its original habitat lies somewhere in the region of east of Caucasus mountains.

Later, Dewey[111,112] states that it probably originated where in Central Asia.

Cannabis seems to have spread to China some 4500 years ago. It progressed spreading to New World during post-Columbian periods. Now it is known in most tropical and temperate lands. It slowly got naturalized in various parts of India and elsewhere, where it occurs as a common weed in wet places.

Plant Cannabis

(a). *Taxonomy*-varieties

Cannabis is one of the most plastic plants ever brought into cultivation, and resulted in the development of at least three distinct types, each of which could be recognised into many varieties, namely one which is grown in Europe, Central Asia and America specifically for exploitation of fibers. The second type is harvested for the fruits and is the source of oil, while the third type flourishes in India, Arabia and North Africa, and is used in the extraction of narcotic products.

These products are derived from the dried inflorescences and upper leaves of the carpellate plants. They produce alkaloids of a narcotic character which are variously termed as 'Ganja', 'Bhang', 'Charas' (in India), Kif (in Algeria and Morrocco), Takrouri (in Tunis), Kabak, Asarath and Nasha (in Turkey), Hashis el Keif (in Syria and Lebanon), Djamba Liamba and Riamba (in Central Africa and Brazil), Dagga (in South Africa), Marihuana (in North America), Suruma (in Mozambique), Rongony (in Malagasy) and Maconhan (in Briasil), Canape (in France), Hanf (in Germany), Konapli (in Italy), Canamo (in Russia), Kanas (in Denmark).

Cannabis sativa Linn. is a true hemp plant cultivated in Europe for its fibers. In general sense the term 'Hemp' means plants producing bast fibers. Doge[115] lists as many as 32 plants having the same name, viz. Manila hemp (leaf stalks of *Musa textiles* Nees), Sisal hemp (Leaves of Agave), Maurtitius hemp (Furcraea gigantea Vent), Sunn hemp (*Crotalaria Juncea* Linn.) etc.

Cannabis is grown for fiber in Russia, throughout Europe, Italy, Africa, India, China, Japan, Brazil, and United States.

Russia produces Cannabis for export, and best fiber quality comes from Italy, mainly due to use of refined process of fiber getting.

In United States it is grown in Wisconsin, Nebrasaka, Kentucky, California, Indiana, and New York (cf. Hayward[115]).

In India, *Cannabis indica* grows wild in waste places in Northern and Western Sub-Himalayas, from Punjab to Bengal, extending southward in Deccan (Ahluwalia[12]).

Family Cannabidaceae

It is a small family, in the order Urticales, earlier included in the family Moraceae (Urticaceae). It contains two genera, namely *Humulus* with 3 species, of which *Humulus lupulis* Linn. is the European hop, while the second is monocarpic *Cannabis*.

Broadly speaking, two species have now been recognised mainly on the basis of products they produce:

(1) *Cannabis sativa* Linn., DC. Prodr., XVI. I, 30. (x = 10, 2n=20-Menzel[234])

(2) Cannabis indica Lamk. (2n=40).

(b) Morphology

Cannabis sativa var. *indica* (syn. *Cannabis indica* Lamk).

Tall, erect, annual herb, 1-5 m. high, all parts with viscid pubescence, monocious, with equal number of male and female plants in single populations. Sometimes dioecious.

Stem angular, sometimes hollow, degree of branching variable, changing with habitat, conditions of cultivation etc.; when grown thickly for fibre production, almost unbranched.

Leaves opposite near the base of them stem, spirally arranged above, stipules small, pointed, persistent, petioles 4-6 cm. long, lamina palmate with 3 to 11 leaflets, upper leaves often with 1leaflet, leaflets sessile, lanceolate, serrate, tip accuminate, green.

Male flowers in axillary and terminal panicles. Female inflorescences, axillary or terminal. Fruit-shining achenes.

Variations

Plant annual, at maturity develops a rigid woody stem, Tall forms are produced in China and Japan, where the slender, sparsely branched stalks have internodes 10-15 cm. long,

The European varieties, usually shorter with more rigid stems, require less time to mature than Asiatic forms.

Shoot : Young stem succulent. At maturity, obtusely hexagonal, more or less furrowed in some varieties hollow.

Heuser[169] reports that cultural conditions exert a great influence on the form of the plant especially with respect to length of the stem and degree of branching.

Watt[322] maintains that with Cannabis indica difference is so marked according to the climate, soil and mode of cultivation, "that we have here in fact, one of the most notable illustrations of the effect of climate in changing the chemical processes, which take place in structure and the physiological peculiarities of a plant."

The phyllotaxy is both opposite and alternate. Schaffner[281,282,283] reports changes of opposite to alternate phyllotaxy as a result of rejuvenation by means of variation in the photoperiod.

Root: It consists of many radiating laterals arising from primary root that extend vertically downward to a variable depth, depending upon the character of the soil.

Heuser[169] observed that roots may even penetrate to a depth of 2 m. in a well-frigated soil, but when plants grow in heavy humus soil, the main tap root, reaches to a maximum of 30-40 cm. depth. The horizontal spread of the laterals depends to a large degree upon the soil type.

Inflorescences: McPhee[227, 228] records that monoecious plants are more common when the daily exposure to light is short and it is possible to modify and control to some degree the product of staminate and carpellate flowers under experimental conditions.

Schaffner[282] data on rejuvenation experiments reveals that sex reversal can be successfully brought about during the second ontogenetic differentiation cycle of rejuvenated plants in individuals that were of pure sex expression in the first or natural differentiation cycle and suggested that "speculations as to nature and fixity of sex, especially in relation to heredity are of questionable value. The formulae based arbitrarily on the behaviour of individual during their first differentiation cycle are not to be accepted as an explanation of the real nature of such individuals". On the other hand, McPhee[228] notes that "Sex determination in *Cannabis* can be explained in a genetic basis and that the inheritance is of the XY type".

Staminate Inflorescence

Staminate flowers develop in small, drooping branched panicles which arise in the axils of foliage leaves.

Flowers of the panicle occur singly on slender pedicles or in groups, usually the terminal branches bear 3 flowers, a median one, and tow laterals, subtended by stipules (bracts).

Individual flowers, apetalous, deeply parted calyx, 5 greenish-yellow lobes, wide-spread at maturity. STamens-5, anthers suspended from thin filaments.

Plants wind pollinated, pollen white, spherical, papilate, liberated through terminal pores.

Sepals oval, acuminate, outer surface and margins covered with multicellular glands, slender, pointed, unicellular hairs, Calcium oxalate deposited in their swollen basis. Stomata present in outer epidermis. Mesophyll spongy 1-2 cells thick.

Ontogeny of the staminate flower has been described by Hayward[155]. According to him the conical floral primordium develops in the axil of a stipule, first produces five cone-shaped initials of the sepals. These arise in a definite succession, the first two are adjacent to the stipule, the third one develops opposite followed by two, placed laterally. After the differentiation of the sepal primordia, the 5 staminal primordia arise, each one being opposite a sepal.

Carpellate Inflorescence

Carpellate flowers are borne in short, compact spikes. Flowers aggregated at the apex of inflorescence, produced in pairs in the axil of leaf. Each flower subtended by a stipule. One of each pair of flowers abortive. Short branches result in formation of compact carpellate inflorescence.

The leaves which sub-tend the paired flower have 2/5 phyllotaxy.

Carpellate flower, simple, consisting of a pistil surrounded by a transparent papery perianth. In normal position, green scabrous floral bract with overlapping edges completely surrounds the mature flower. It is conical, open at the top, terminated by a beak, when uncurled and expanded, heart-shaped and acuminate. Abaxial surface of the bract thickly covered with glands and glandular emergences, intermixed with large, stout conical hairs. Abaxial surface devoid of glands, hairs present at the margin near the apex of the bract where the inner surface is more exposed.

Perianth continuous, entire, cupshaped, smooth to slightly friged margin, at maturity covers 2/3 of ovary.

Perianth, simple hyaline, membranous, consisting of two epidermal layers between which are a few spongy mesophyll cells. Cells of the abaxial epidermis elongated in the direction of the long axis of the ovary. Adaxial surface resembles the abaxial one. It is devoid of hairs. Mesophyll composed of transparent, thin-walled cells, homogeneous, non-chlorophyllose, 3 to 4 cells thick.

Pistil, oval, unilocular, slightly flattened, somewhat depressed at its stylar ends. Two stylar branches and atigmas. Styles, cylindrical, papillate stigmas.

Briosi and Tognini[67] states that the primordium of the carpellate flower originates as a dome-shaped structure in the axil of a foliar bract or stipule.

At the base of the flower there is a floral bract. Ovary wall arises as a ring-like fold at the base of the floral primordium and gradually encloses its apex. When the ovary walls gets completely overgrown the floral axis, two opposing points on its margin begin to grow more rapidly initiating the two styles and stigmas. The styles elongate unequally.

Within the ovary, the remaining tissue of the primordium forms the nucellus, and finally a single ovule is developed which becomes completely campylotropous with a curved mega-gametophyte.

Briosi and Tognini[67] records knob-like projections at the base of the ovary and above the perianth. These have been interpreted by them, as being rudimentary primordia of stamens in which development has been arrested.

Zinger[345] described the ontogeny of the carpellate flower little different than the description given above as recorded by Hayward[155]. In most of the varieties of *Cannabis* examined, by found that there were two distinct perianth primordia. The first primordium appears at the base of the floral axis on the side towards the floral bract, while the second develops on the dorsal side of the floral axis at a higher level than the first. Both are not perceptible until the carpellary primordia are differentiated.

Zinger[345] found perianth completely enclosing the basal portion of the ovary in two horticultural varieties which he designated as *Cannabis gigantea* Hort. and *C. Himalayana* Hort.

Zinger[345] noticed that the massive inner integument becomes completely coalescent with the thick outer one, and covers the apex of the nucellus in such a way that the micropylar canal becomes closed by the integumentary issue. After pollination, the pollen tube either grows through the tissue which fills the micropyle or penetrates the two integuments, on reaching nucellus, branches at the apex then sends single branch into the megagametophyte.

Embryology

After fertilization, transverse segmentation of the zygote produces the suspensor and embryo proper. The suspensor remains as a short stalk one–two cells thick. Embryo is at first globular, but there is an early differentiation of the cotyledons which develop as lateral lobes on either side of the growing point of the epicotyl.

Concurrent with the development of the embryo, an abundant endosperm is formed which fills the embryo sac. This is gradually utilized by the embryo. Savelli[278] reports presence of twin embryos.

Microscopy of the Fruit and Seed

Fruit is an achene light brown-grey-brown in colour, sometimes mottled. It is smooth, compressed, orbicular to oval in shape and varies in size.

Heuser[169] reports that the average length of the European species varies from 4.3 mm. diameters to 2.75-3.3 mm. dewey[111] on the other hand records the length of the fruit varying from 3 to 6 mm. with diameters 2.5 to 4 mm.

The 'seed' of commerce is actually the fruit, which in some cases comes into market enclosed within its hooded floral bract.

The outer epidermis of the floral bract is characterized by presence of hair and glands.

Hair reach a length of 0.5 to 1.0 mm. tapering at an apex and spherical at base. The globular gland consists of eight or more cells radiating from two central ones, which are sessile, sometimes they are borne on many-celled stalks.

The pericarp of the fruit, is composed of 5 distinct regions. (The outermost layer or epicarp is made up of sclerenchymatous cells, sinuous in outline in surface view). Radially their walls are slightly thickened at some regions, while in other they become thick as to narrow down the lumen of the cell. All the layers are porous. The second region is spongy parenchyma, consisting of one to many layers of colourless cells with interpolating various intercellular spaces.

Epicarp shows numerous anastomosing bundles and which gets thickened along the two keels of the fruit.

The third zone is formed of hypodermal layers of brown contents and thick walls. The fourth layer consists of small, colourless, porous, dwarf cells with sinuous radial walls.

The innermost zone of the pericarp consists of palisade cells with thick outer and radial walls.

The seed coat consists of two distinct layers. Outer-most comprising of tube cells, while inner layer consists of irregular parenchymatous cells.

In mature fruit, the periperm and endosperm are each, one cells layer in thickness, and adhere to each other.

Endosperm extends as a membrane between cotyledons and hypocotyl. It is several layers in thickness.

The cells of the endosperm contain protein grains.

The embryo is curved with its axis U-Shaped, consists of two plano-convex cotyledons, enclosing a well-developed epicotyl, a sub-cylindrical hypocotyl and primary root. Epidermal layers of the cotyledons are composed of small cells containing aleurone grains.

Below the abaxial epidermis are many layers of isodiametric cells, while beneath the adaxial portion lies 2-many layers of palisade cells. The embryo lies with tip of primary root and apices of the cotyledons directed towards micropylar (chalazal) end of the seed.

Development and Ontogeny

The development of the seedling has been fully described by Hayward[155] and some important points are recorded here.

At germination, primary root emerges from fruit coat at stylar end, splitting the coat, into two. Primary tap root grows at the rate of 7.5-10.0 cm. within 48 hours after emergence. One the 4th day lateral roots develop. By this time hypocotyl also elongates and becomes erect. Epicotyl is pubescent increasing slightly in diameter towards the cotyledonary node. Expansion of cotyledons is rapid on their setting free from fruit coat.

Lubbock[213] records various sizes, namely ones ranging from 1.4-1.6 cm. while the other 1.0-1.3 cm. long.

For the first 15-20 days cotyledons carry out photosynthetic function as well as act as storage organ, later they get discoloured and wither away.

Cotyledons-obvate to spatulate, tapers toward bases, terminal portions recurved. They are sessile, connate at base, forming cotyledonary collar. Venation consists of a prominent midrib with two-lateral veins, arising from its base which unite with other two, originating from midvein at the midpoint of the cotyledon.

Lamina of cotyledon-thick spongy then first foliage leaves.

Mesophyll-chlorophyllose 2-3 layer of palisade cells. Adaxial portion of leaf contain 2-3 layers. Abaxial 10- many layers.

Stomata occur on upper and lower epidermis. Both surfaces covered with unicellular hair.

Berkman[44] noticed that first internode reaches its normal length of 3-5 cm. by 12-13th day.

The first pair of foliage leaves above cotyledons are simple, ovate with serrate margins.

In most instances, the second and the third pairs are digitate, the former usually having three leaflets and the latter four or five.

Histological Characteristics

Root: is diarch with two groups of primary pholem flanking the primary xylem strand.

Protoxylem abuts the pericycle, which is multiseriate, consisting of 4 to many layers, laying centrally, In intercotyledonary plane it is usually two layers in width. Endodermis is uniseriate, casparian strips begin to differentiate at about the time when metazylem matures. Cortex composes of

5-7 cocentric layer of parenchymatous cells with intercellular spaces. Outer layers form a distinct hypodermis.

Root shows cone-shaped, blunt root cap.

There are different views regarding the structure and ontogeny of the root.

Van Tieghem and Douliot[307] records pericycle to be a single layer of cells and interprets periblem to be a layer of initials.

Flahault[134], Briosi and Tognini[68] and Berkman[44] found that the periblem consists of two layers of initials and the pericyclic layer changes into multiseriate layer as a result of periclinal divisions.

In the ontogeny of the root, the primary structures are derived from three well-defined histogens which are similar to those described by Janczewski[180] and Crooks[102].

The root cap and epidermis are derived from a common layer of initials-calyptrogendermatogen. The cortical tissue originate from the two layered periblem, and the stelar tissues are derived from the plerome.

The development of the root cap and epidermis from the calyptrogen-dermatogen layer results from the differential character of the division of its cells. The cells of this layer which immediately overlie the periblem at the tip of the root divide periclinally to form the root cap cells. The more laterally placed ones divide anti-climally, and function as a true dermatogen in producing the epidermis.

The manner in which root cap and dermatogen arise from the dual histogen has been fully described by de Bary[39].

The cortex is derived from two-layered periblem; it forms a terminal cap over group of plerome cells at the root apex. The outer layer of the periblem divides only in anticlinal planes, thus giving rise to the outermost cortical layer which become the hypodermis.

The initials of the inner layer divide in all planes to produce 4-7 layered parenchymatous cortex and the endodermis.

The pericycle is the first tissue of the stele to differentiate, being derived from the outermost layer of the plerome. With differentiation of the pericycle, the primary pholem and xylem develops simultaneously.

The protophloem comprises of elongated parenchymatous cells with small diameters. The primary phloem ducts are formed by the breakdown of the linear row of cells adjacent to the pericycle, 3 to 4 groups occur in each phloem strand.

Primary xylem consists of 3-5 thin-walled annular and spiral elements, constituting each protoxylem group. The outermost, the smallest abuts the inner layer of pericycle and is 3-4 cells in width by the time the first annular vessels mature.

The metaxylem elements mature centripetally. They have bordered pits with narrow thin torus.

de Litardiere[208] and Breslawetz[61] reports tetraploidy in the primary root. The diploid number of chromosomes in *Cannabis* is 20 and this is seen in the cells of the plerome, but both investigators found tetraploid of 40 in the cells of periblem. This observation was made by de Litardiere[208] in specimens collected from two different varieties of *Cannabis* grown in different localities and his results were confirmed by observations of Breslawetz[61]. This means this condition is general, rather than aberrant. Several explanations have been put forth. Breslawetz[61] suggests it is due to the occurrence of nuclear divisions in the cells of the periblem which is not succeeded by cytogenesis, but by the enlargement of the cells involved and by fusion of the two nuclei in each cell.

de Litardiere[208] on the other hand, did not observe any binucleate cells and suggests that the situation may arise from anormal metaphase, followed by a monocentric telephase which would produce a single tetraploid daughter nucleus.

The Stem

The fibre of commerce is derived from the stem, and consequently its structure has been extensively studied by textile engineers.

Dewey[111, 112] reports that the ideal plant in terms of exploitation is the one which attains a height of 10-12 ft., Ō–3/8" in diameter at the base, and develops internodes 10 or more inches in length. Stem should be fluted, with comparatively large central cavity so it is easily broken during retting.

The young stem is grooved and ridged, owing to development of principal bundles and the longitudinal strands of collenchyma. These are arranged in a ring and are separated from one another by medullary rays, which are later occuluded with an inter fascicular cambium, which develops and secondary growth begins.

Epidermis–cutinized, with numerous hair and glands There are 2 types of hair (i) pointed non-glandular, unicellular hair which develop from raised base, sometimes break off leaving warty circular scars. Cystoliths are found in the bases of epidermal hair produced on the leaves and floral bracts. (ii) glandular, multicellular hair. Stomata present.

Heuser[169] records stomatal frequency 12 per sq. cm. But Briosi and Tognini[67, 68] reports 5 per sq. mm. in young stem having 2 mm. diameter, pointing out that the frequency per unit area diminishes greatly as the stem matures.

Radial and tangential diameters of the epidermal cells are approximately equal, and they are 3 to 4 times as long as broad.

Below the epidermis lies chlorenchymatous zone, 2-3 cells wide, extends completely around the periphery of the stem including the ridges where it separates the collenchyma from the epidermis.

This chlorenchymatous layer is compact in very young stems but get tangentially stretched and develop large intercellular spaces.

Hypodermal layer consists of larger cells and they are much thickened. At ridges compact collenchymatous cells are found within the zone of chlorenchyma.

Cortex consists of a few layers of parenchymatous cells. In old stems pericycle is multilayered, in which fibre develops. There cells can be distinguished in transactions of a relative young stem, as they form a definite zone of angular cells lying between the phloem and cortex.

Collateral vascular bundles are separated from one another by medullary rays. The number of primary bundles varies at different stem levels, owing to branching and anatomoses, an varies from a 2/5 spiral to a decussate phyllotaxy.

Briosi and Tognini[68] traced the course and number of bundles of the stem axis beginning in the hypocotyl.

At each successive branch, the hypo-cotyledonary bundle increase from 2 to 4, 8 to 12, then anatomose reducing to 10. of these 4 comprise the cotyledonary traces and enter the cotyledons at the cotyledonary node. At every succeeding internode the number of primary bundles range from 12 to 16, depending upon the location of the transaction examined in relation to a node.

Three bundles supply each leaf. Primary xylem consists of

annular, spiral reticulate and pitted vessels. Xylem fibres do not exceed 0.5 mm. and are uniform in length.

Phloem consists of sieve tubes, companion cells, parenchyma fibres and resin ducts. Sieve tubes have transverse or oblique sieve plates. Companion cells slender and tapering. Phloem fibres small, short, thin-walled. They occur in zones in the pholem singly or in groups.

In older steams secondary growth results in successive zones of fibres, giving phloem a banded appearance.

Zander[343] has described the structure and development of the ducts in details and states that they are unbranched, unicellular and multinucleate. They are absent in root and cotyledons.

Ducts contain golden-brown granular substance and large spindle-shaped nuclei.

The ducts extended through more than one internode of a mature plant exceed to about 30 cm. or more in length. They occur in the outer limits of the primary pholem, and number of ducts in transactions of stems, vary in age from very young seedlings to mature plants.

Pith consists of large thin-walled cells with inter cellular spaces.

Percyclic Fibres

Bredemann[60] and Heuser[169] point out that staminate plants produce fibres of better quality than the carpellate ones, and despite the fact that the number of carpellate ones, and despite the fact that the number of carpellate plants slightly exceeds the staminate in a given crop, the percentage of fibre-content, is greater for the staminate plants than for the carpellate ones.

Ontogenic studies reveal that pericyclic cells enlarge, elongate, become vacuoalte and the cytoplasm finally forms a thin layer against the primary wall. As secondary wall formation continues, lumen of each fiber becomes smaller, cytoplasm concentrates. At maturity within the fiber, cytoplasm disintegrates leaving an elongated oval lumen.

Italian *Cannabis* are found to contain 77.77% of cellulose. It exhibits stratification.

Structure of the Fiber

Mathews[224] in his study on textile fibers records that a

single *Cannabis* fiber is 3-7 angled in cross-section. It later gets compressed in old stems, where secondary growth takes place, the angles become rounded or even flattened.

Average diameter is 22 m, but one finds great variation between individual fibers, greatest diameter reached has been from 16-50 m as reported by Cross and Bevan[103].

The diameter of a given fiber is very variable, as fiber tapers at both ends, the range of length is from 1 to 10 cm. Heuser[169] records average length between 3-5-4 cm.

The tips of the fiber cells are rounded to blunt, sometimes forked and this is one of the diagnostic characters of separating northern and southern varieties of hemp, in which later varieties show prominent forking. Schilling[280] has noticed that bifurcation of fiber could be experimentally induced by mechanical means.

Leaf

Lamina is thin, with principal veins forming prominent ridges on abaxial surface.

Adaxial surface depressed into a groove above each vein.

The cells of upper epidermis larger and more cutinized then of the lower ones. Stomata prominent on lower surface.

Briosi and Tognini[68] records the following observations of various parts.

Number of stomata per sq.mm. on cotyledons –100 (upper and lower epidermis). Central leaflet 350, Foliar bract 700. Stipule 55. Sepal of staminate flower 100. Floral bract 43.

Epidermal hair are produced on both surfaces.

Mesophyll consists of a single layer of slender, lonaged palisade cells. Spongy parenchyma with large intercellular spaces leading to sub-stomatal cavities. Midvein of the leaflet reinforced by a group of mechanical cells, located below the groove on the adaxial surface.

Vascular bundle collateral. Latex ducts occur in primary phloem and extend into the stem without branching.

Newer Facts About the Plant

1. Cultivation

In India the total area under ganja is as follows: Bihar -65 hectares, Hyderabad—prohibited, Madhya Pradesh—17 h., Mysore— prohibited, Manipur—prohibited, Orissa—5h., W. Bengal—36 h.

Cultivation is done under Government license.

Mikuriya[237] states that 'Kif' (*Cannabissativa*) is the main cash crop of Rif Mountains. It yields marketable product of dried stem, tops up to 2 kg./sq. mm.

Breeding for Fibres

Antoniani[28] experimented on new *Cannabis* varieties in Emilia. He states that on comparison of German *Cannabis* varieties–Elite 55, Super Elite 56 (Fibranova) and Fibridia with Italian variety–Carmagnola, he found that they were less vigorous, showed earlier maturity, less resistance to wind and to broomrape infestation showed lower stem yield and lower fibre quality, but the fibre yield per ha. were considerably higher than with Carmagnola. All these varieties were economically superior to the Italian variety Fibranova. The optimal density for all varieties was 125 plants per sq. m. but, with closer spacing adopted for the improvement of fibre quality, the response was greater in the German, than in Italian types. The new varieties showed a better response than Carmagnola to Nitrogen up to 120 kg./ha. but heavier applications increased the tendency to lodging. Foliar applications of urea had no effect on yield and only slightly extended the growing period. In the second year tests fibre quality was higher in Fibranova than in Carmagnola. Irrigation, even in a dry season, was of no advantage on the good soils, and Nitrogen proved slightly detrimental. Ins some instances Elite 55 proved superior in production and quality to Fibranova variety.

Jeung Haeng Ree[183] describes the growing of *Cannabis* in Korea, as a major fibre crop. He records that it is grown on both upland and paddy lands. he describes cultural practices followed. Further he points out that the yield per unit area is not satisfactory, but can be increased by improving the present fertilizer practices and replacing the local variety with higher yielding Japanese variety–Tochiker or a hybrid of this and a local variety.

Allavena[15] points out the advantages of Bredemann's method for determination of fibre yield in *Cannabis* for purpose of selection.

The characteristic features of the method are: (i) separation of primary from secondary fibres, and (ii) chemical maceration to obtain pure fibres. Its adoption led to breeding of the new variety Fibranova, which has a high fibre content.

Allavena[16] further traces the new developments in *Cannabis* growing in Italy. He records that a new variety of Fibranova has been evolved and is replacing variety Carmagnola.

Bocsa and Farkas[52] experimented with the scion of *Cannabis* and carried out longevity grafting trials with the rootstock.

Scions taken from varieties with a relatively long growing season prolonged the life of the rootstocks of varieties with a shorter growing season.

Scions from female plants took longer growing period than male plants.

Nevinnyh[246] carried out breeding and selection experiments. He found that the first generation hybrids after crossing a dioecious female parent with a monoecious variety were predominantly female, nut lack crossing the first generation hybrid with a monoecious variety resulted in an increase in the number of monoecious hybrids which was maintained in subsequent generations. Early ripening, higher yields and increased vigour were dominant characteristics of the hybrids. Fibre yields were either midway between those of the parent plants or similar to those of the less fibrous of the parents.

Szilagyi[302] records production of tetraploid *Cannabis* by treatment of germination seedlings with 0.05 percent colchicine.

Spladon, Laskos and Vasuta[289] investigated the trials on seed rates of *Cannabis* variety Ratislavicke sown in rows 60 cm. apart at 10, 17.5 and 25 kg./ha. with a fourth treatment consisting of thinning to 60 x 60 cm. with 2-3 plants per group. Row distances were kept at a standard rate of 20 kg/ha. Seeds were sown 50, 60 and 70 cm. apart. The highest seed yields were obtained from thinning to 60 x 60 cm. and from using a row distance of 70 cm. The latter being the most economical methods of cultivation.

Tudosie and Topor[316] cultured hemp for special purpose, namely for producing twine for use in vine yards and rootstock nurseries. They found use of *Cannabis* instead of raffia or strips of lime bark greatly reduces the cost of production.

2. Ecology

Cannabis can be grown over a great range of altitudes, climates and soils. The best development of fibre is in mild humid climates of the temperate regions with the temperatures of 60-80°F cularly for germination and establishment, and on rich loamy soils.

For the production of narcotics or narcotic resin, hotter more tropical conditions are required. Sex expression is altered by environmental conditions, particularly the length of the day, short days favouring monoecious conditions. (Purseglove[261]).

Schaffner[281] investigated the various hereditary expressions in *Cannabis sativa* induced by changed ecological conditions, especially twisting and twining of the hypocotyle, development at maturity of only 2-4 internodes instead of 20-40, change of leaf arrangement from opposite to alternate, development of peculiar types of sexual dimorphism, change of sexual expression from unisexuality to bisexuality, production of 4 blooming periods instead of the usual 1, expression of peculiar types of leaves through rejuvenation, in the rejuvenation zone, flower development on the petiole.

From his experiments he found that the definition of the heredity should be changed. According to him, heredity is an expression or repetition from generation to generation from time to time, of the characteristics of an organism as determined by a given set of definite, self perpetuating protoplasmic units and by a given complex of definite environmental conditions.

There are always two general factors in the equation which determines the given expression, the protoplasmic mechanism and the ecological condition.

A change of the proper magnitude in either results in a change of character. The environment has potentiality as well as protoplast. The protoplasmic units or autogens perpetuate themselves by assimilation and division.

Lacznska-Hulewicowa[200] in his experiments on the effects of external factors on the sex of *Cannabis* records that when diploid and tetraploid *Cannabis sativa* was sown in pots and the fields on various dates and given various photoperiodic treatments. The day length had a definite effect on sex expression in tetraploid *Cannabis* especially in monecious plants.

Short days (10 hours) induced the development of female

sex characters and increased the size of somatic cells, and though not altering the size of the pollen grains, retarded the development of the stamens and pollen. On changing over to long days, normal viable pollen was formed.

When the changeover from short to long days was abrupt the plants, especially the tetraploids, became deformed and the formation of floral organs was often disrupted.

3. Production and Utilization

Ashe[32] has given very comprehensive details about hem production and utilization in United States. She states that United states' annual production of the formerly very important bast fibre has fallen from about 75,000 tons, a century ago, to about 2000 tons today. Imports too have dropped. Other fibres, particularly abaca, have replaced it more and more.

Hopkins[174] has produced another memoir on the hemp industry in Kentucky; in it he writes that in the colonial days of America and the first 80 years of succeeding new Republic, while sailing vessels were in vogue, hemp fibre was a commodity of importance, for it was the material out of which sails and cordage for shipping was made. Kentucky became one of the principal hemp-producing states.

In 1810, Kentucky contributed all the hemp imported three-fourths of the crops of 1840, one-half of the yield in 1847, and in 1849 and about one third the total production of 1859.

The largest producer of Cannabis today, is the Soviet Union with an annual production approximately nearing 115,000 tons compared with the estimated world production (excluding China) of 280,000 tons.

The principal exporting countries are Italy, and Yugoslavia and the principal importing countries are West Germany and France. Outside Europe, *Cannabis* is produced commercially in China, Japan, Chile and Peru.

Increased production occurred in the United States during World Warr II. (Purseglove[261]).

4. Physiology

Arnouz[31] found that *Cannabis* is a short day plant, in a photoperodic cycle including a long night, the production of male flowers was inhibited and the number of female phenotypes increased. The variety Fibrimon-56 was most sensitive to short days during the period from 10th to 20th day of growth; in the variety 0.63 the most sensitive period was from the 20th to the 30th day of growth.

Atal[33] observed that a weekly application of a 100 ppm. GA spray to young *Cannabis sativa* plants increased stem and internode length, fresh and dry weight of the stem, the bark, wood ratio and number of fibres, suppressed lateral branching and root development. Individual fibre of treated plants was upto 10 times longer, more lignified and had larger diameter than those of untreated plants, and it is considered that G.A. treatment may prove to be of commercial importance.

Cajlahjan, Kocankov and Zamota[76] investigated the effect of gibberellin on the growth and yield of *Cannabis* and tobacco.

They found in their container experiments that 5 spray applications of .0001-0.01.% GA to *Cannabis* and 6 applications to tobacco increased the height of both plants 2Ū times, and their fresh weight almost as much and doubled the number of tobacco leaves.

In *Cannabis* the treatment increased the fibre content and size of the staple and reduced the time required for retting.

Davidjan[105, 106] experiment increased the fibre content and the size of the staple and reduced the time required for retting.

Davidjan[105, 106] experimented with the growth and development of *Cannabis* in relation to light conditions. He found that plants from north, south and central Russia were grown under photoperiods ranging from 8 to 16 hours for 50 days, followed by transfer to natural days.

Growth was depressed as the length of the photoperiod decreased. Under 14 and 16 hours days the growth of varieties from northern and Central Russia was depressed more than that of the southern variety, but under 8, 10 and 12 hour days the reverse was true.

Under natural-day conditions the plants did not branch, but when short days were followed by natural day treatment the central Russian and southern varieties produced side-shoots. Shortday treatment accelerated flowering in plants were also noted.

Davidjan[106] further investigated the growth of the root system of *Cannabis* in relation to day length. He found that in southern and the northern *Cannabis* variety the total length and the general vigour of the roots and the height of the stem were greater when grown in natural than in 10-hour day lengths. During the early developmental stages the roots grew more vigorously than the stem, but at the stage of intensive development (from the beginning of bud formation to flowering), the growth of both roots and stems greatly increased. During that period, in natural day length, root growth in the southern variety reached a maximum daily average of 8 cm. The female plants had a more vigorous root system that the male.

Herich[165] found that both quantitative and qualitative changes occurred in 13 free aminoacids and amides of *Cannabis* seeds treated with GZ at 10 to 200 ppm.

Janisevskij[180, 181] noticed pot grown *Cannabis* seedlings of the variety Ju S-I were sprayed 3 times with 0.01 percent G.A.. The treatment promoted stem extension and slightly increased the fresh weight of the plants, but slightly decreased their dry weight.

In the treated plants the chlorophyll, total Nitrogen and protein Nitrogen were reduced, but soluble N was increased. A decrease observed in the nucleic acid content was mainly due to a reduction of RMA. Practically no change occurred in the N fractions of the nuclei and plastida.

Kalinkevic and Udovenko[186] studied the effects of $Ca(No_3)_2$, NH_4OH, $NH_4OH + KCL$, NH_4CL and $(NH_4)_2SO_4$ on the contents of 17 aminoacids in the stems of pot grown *Cannabis* plants.

Lalakis[203] was able to attain polyploids from *Cannabis sativa* by application of colchicine. He followed the following procedures:

The tips of one-week old seedlings of *Cannabis* were immersed for 3 hours in a 0.5% colchicine solution and this solution was found to be more effective in inducing polyploidy than soaking of seeds or immersing seelings. The treated plants become tetraploid and produce triploid progenies when crossed with the parent type.

About 90% of these triploid plants were monoecious and declinous.

Lesik[204] observed the effects of form by nitrogen fertilizers on carbohydrate-protein metabolism of *Cannabis*.

He found that fertilizers applied to *Cannabis* plants contained nitrogen in any one of the three forms namely ammonium nitrate, sodium nitrate or ammonium sulphate. The NH_4 fertilizers produced higher concentrations of proteins and sugars in the leaves. This was associated with a higher concentration of cellulose an d a lower concentration of pectins in the fibres, causing on improvement in their quality.

Paskovic[256] in glass house experiments sprayed *Cannabis* with GA at 1, 10 and 100 mg/1. when the plants were 20, 40, 50 cm. high. Rates of 10 and 100 mg./1. applied on either of the first two dates increased stem height, but 1 mg./1. reduced it.

Plants grown from seeds treated with 1 and 100 mg/1. G.A. were smaller, but those treated with 10 mg/1. were larger than the controls. All the sprayed plants had a tender sickly appearance.

Sudi[298] experimented on seeds treated with 3, 5 dichlorophenoxyacetic acid (3,5-U), 3-5-dichloro-phenoxy-acetamide (3, 5-D-Am.) and its N-methyl-, N-ethyl and N-but). derivatives (35 D-Me, 35 D-Et and 35 D-Bu respectively). The response of the seedlings, based on the degree of swelling was found to be weak when treated with 35 D-Bu.

All substances used inhibited growth at 100 ppm., while others at 10 ppm. and the effect increased with increasing concentration.

5. Flower, Sex Expression

Conrad[98, 99] noticed that during flowering male stems and leaves contained larger amounts of growth substances than female stems and leaves. Higher contents of growth substances were found in withering stems and leaves.

Heslop-Harrison[168] records the suppressive effects of 2-thouracil on differentiation and flowering of *Cannabis sativa*. He found that the pyrimidine, 2-thiouracil, partly annuls the effect of photo-periodic induction in the short day plant, when it is supplied at the onset of the dark period in quantities of 15-30 ug. per plant. This treatment also produces aberrations in cellular differentiation in the leaves. Tracer studies show that 2-thirouracil becomes bound in cellular ribonucleic acid, which suggests that the effects on morphogenesis are due to interference with nucleic acid metabolism.

Laskowska[202] investigated the influence of the age of pollen and stigmas on sex determination in *Cannabis*. The results of pollination of stigmas of different ages with pollen which had been stored for different periods are tabulated in terms of the sex ratios of subsequent generations. The age of the stigma was without influence on sex determination. Pollen up to 6 hours old and also 14-17 days old, caused a predominance of female plants in the first and second generations. Pollen 12 and 24 hours old did not change the sex ratio.

6. Sex Differentiation

Bocsa[52] found that on crossing a special mompecious hybrid bred by the author with various dioecious strains, F hybrids were obtained with 93.4 percent unisexual plants of which 60.7 per cent were pure females and 30.7 percent monoecious. The maximum percentage of unisexual plants produced was 97.9 percent. The hybrid yielded 70.5 percent more seeds than the dioecious mother strain. This was due entirely to the increase in functionary female flowers, since the yielding capacity and the seed weight of the individual hybrid plants were lower than in the parent.

Conrad and Mothers[98] studied the sex-link differences in auxin content of dioecious *Cannabis*. He found that auxin content (IAA equivalent per Kg. of fresh weight) was 6 and 8 in male plants as compared with 180 and 220 in female plants.

Herich[160, 161] investigated the problem of sex differentiation in *Cannabis*. He found that by soaking the seeds of the hemp variety polyploidna in solutions of $Mn\ So_4$, KBr, K.I. or H_2O_2 the percentage of female plants were reduced and that of male and monoecious plants increased. In the variety 'sumperska' seed treatment also reduced the percentage of female plants and increased that of male plants.

Furthermore, he observed the effect of boron on the process of sex differentiation. Soaking of the seeds of two hemp varieties in 0.2 and 0.5 percent $H_3\ BO_3$ gave similar results as those obtained with $Mn\ SO_4$.

Herich[162, 165] noticed that when the seeds are soaked for 24 hours in solutions containing 5, 10, 25 and 100 ppm. of GA, the percentage of female individual increased, the highest increase being caused by the 10 ppm. concentration. When the average stem lengths were compared at the end of the vegetative growth, the greatest response was shown by female plants treated by 5 ppm., the optimum for males being 10 ppm. The inhibiting effects of higher concentrations were most marked with female plants.

Heslop-Harrison[167] experimented upon temperature-induced meristematic and other variations in *Cannabis sativa*.

He found that when photoperiods inducing rapid flowering were combined with low night temperature, a high proportion of the flowers became inter-sexual. Intersexuality in male flowers involved a transformation of stamens to carpellate or intermediate structures.

Kohler[193] noticed that the genetic factors could be effected by different photoperiods.

Limberk[207] studied the influence of photoperiodicity on the sexual index in *Cannabis*.

He found that when plants were sown at intervals from november to august, male plants usually flowered earlier than females.

In april, when the day length exceeded 14 hours, the female plants ceased to flower and continued vegetative growth, but began to flower again in august when the day length had dropped to about 15 hours.

Male plants flowered even during the longest days. A reduction in the light intensity by shading increased the proportion of female plants, particularly if the shading was imposed in 2-3 weeks after germination.

Intersexual plants were observed only during the short day (11-13 hr.) period.

Zemljanuhin and Sensina[344] found that in staminate plants, during the flowering stage the respiration rate, organic phosphate, sucrose contents and ascorpinoxidase activity were higher than in pistillate plants, where as in the latter the total P and ascorbic acid contents and the reducing capacity were higher.

Pre-sowing seed treatments with ascorbic, succinic, aspartic acids and cystine increased the pistillate characteristics, while X-rays treatment tended to intensify the staminate features, but CO had no effect no sex expression.

7. Embryology

Briosi and Tongnini[67], Davis[109], Elfving[121], MacPhee[227], Tournois[312, 313], Wettstein[328, 329], Winge[330], and Zinger[345] investigated the embryology of *Cannabis*. They state another of Cannabiaceae as a whole is tetrasporangiate with a cutinized epidermis. But in *Cannabis sativa* endothecial cells are filled with resin, two or three middle layers are ephemeral, cells of glandular tapetum 2-nucleate. Cytokinesis in the microspore follows meiosis. Microspore tetrad, tetrahedral. Pollen grains, 2-celled.

Ovule anatropous, bitegmic, crassinuclellar with micropyle formed by inner integument. Archesporial cell cuts off a primary parietal cell which gives rise to 7 parietal layers, an d the apical cells of the nucellar epidermis divide periclinally to form a nucellar cap 2 cells in thickness. Cytokinesis in the megaspore mother cells accompanies meiosis and the chalazal megaspore of a linear tetrad develops into a Polygonum type embryo sac. The synergids are short pyriform, polar nuclei fuse before fertilization, and the 3 antipodal cells are ephemeral.

Apomixis has been suspected in *C. Sativa* and *Humulus lupulus* (Strasburger[297]).

Endosperm formation is nuclear and during early post fertilization stages, the base of the embryo sac elongates in a curved manner and becomes haustorial. Wall formation is initiated around the globular embryo. Endosperm becomes cellular, except for the chalazal haustorium, remains coenocytic until collapse.

Embryogeny is of onagrad type. In. *C. sativa,* suspensor 2-celled. Poly-embryony is of occasional occurrence in *Cannabis*.

8. Chromosomes

Menzel[234] studied meiotic chromosomes of monoecious Kentucky hemp (*Cannabis sativa*), wherein he records that monoecious plants of hemp were characterized by the absence and dioecious plants by the presence of the heteromorphic pair of chromosomes.

Cannabis sativa L. (X=10, 2n=20).

9. Pollination

The flowers of Cannabis are wind pollinated.

10. Endosperm

Ram[264] was the first to point out the occurrence of endosperm haustorium in *Cannabis sativa* Linn.

11. Germination

The seeds germinate at low temperatures but not below 1°C. Healthy seeds give 90 percent germination and remain viable for at least 2 years if properly stored.

12. Seed Oil

The plants remaining in the field after harvesting for fibre are allowed to set seeds. They are cut when fruits ripen and threshed for seed collection. 1,200-1500 lbs. of seeds are yielded per acre.

Cannabis seeds are fruits in true sense, round to ovate in shape with oily sweet taste. The average composition of the seeds are as follows:

Water-8.75% protein-21.51% fat—30.41%.

N-free extract—15.89%, FibreΔ—18.84%, Ash—4.6%.

A crystalline globulin, edestin has been isolated from defeated meal. It has the following amino acid composition:

Glycocoll-3.8%, Alanine-3.6%, Valine + leucine = 20.9%, Phenylalanine-2.4%, Tryrosine-2.13%, Serine-0.33%, Cystine-0.25%, Proline-4.1%, Oxyproline-2.0%, Aspartic acid-4.5%, Glutamic acid-18.74%, trytophane + arginine-14.36%, lysine-1.67% and histidine-2.36% (cf. Wealth of India 1960).

The seeds yield by expression 32-35 percent of a greenish yellow drying oil with the following characteristics: Sp. gr.$^{15.5^\circ}$, 0.0.925-0.933, sap val 190-195, iod, val. 140-166, and titer. Val. 14-17°. The component fatty acids are Oleic-15%, linolic-70%, linolenic and isolinolenic acids 15%.

Cannabis seed oil is used in paints and varnishes frequently as a substitute for linseed oil and in the manufacture of soft soaps. It is also an excellent medium for grinding colours.

The seed cake, which is used in India s cattle feed, shows following average composition.

Moisture-10.81%, Fat-10.17%, Protein-30.76%, N-free extract-40.59% and ash-7.67%. The mineral constituents of the ash are: K_2O-20.28%, Na_2O-0.78%, CaO-23.64%, MgO-5.70% FE_2O_3-1.00% Mn_2O_3-trace, P_2O_5-36.46%, SO_3-0.19%, SiO_2-11.90%, Cl-P.08% (Winton and Winton[331]).

Cannabis seeds are also used as bird and poultry feed.

13. Commercial Fibers

(i) *Retting and Stripping*: The decline in hemp production in Northern Italy is attributed to the lack of labour for hand retting and stripping. A pilot factory has proved that in 2-6 days a product as good as that from hand operations requiring 5-9 days can be produced by machinery, which removes 50 per cent of the stem materials before the rest is retted. *Clostridium* species are used in the retting tanks. (C-C[89]).

(ii) *Fibre*: Cannabis fibre is strong, lustrous and durable. Commercial fibre is 40-80 inches in length. Finenes of staple is less than that of linen, though its tensile strength is appreciably greater. Microscopically, fibre is seen to consist of cell elements which are unusually long, averaging about 0.73 inch in length and 22" in diameter. The fibre ends are bluntly rounded. The fibre is somewhat uneven in diameter and exhibits frequent longitudinal fractures and swollen fissures. It is made up of a mixture of cellulose and lignocellulose. Chemical analysis of *Cannabis* fibre shows: Water (hygroscopic)-8.88%, Ash-0.82%, Fat- and wax-0.56% aq. extract-3.4%, Cellulose-77.77%, and intercellular matter and pectin bodies-93.31%.

Hemp is used in the manufacture of fine cordage, twine, sailcloth, tarpaulins and carpet yarns. Loose fibre is used for caulking boats, pumps, engines and other machinery.

During the Second World War green fibre prepared without getting by a process of decoricating and cottonising, was used as substitute for jute in making binder twine and sacks. The sue of hemp in cordages, twines and ropes has declined, its place being taken by the hard fibres i.e. Manila and Sisal. Hemp stems can be used for the manufacture of coarse paper (F.A.O. World Fibre Survey 131, 1947).

(iii) *Newer Investigations*: Bellini[43] studied the changes in the fibre content of Carmagnola variety and found the fibres in the basal internodes of 40-days old *Cannabis* plants. In the male plants the percentage fibre content reached a maximum 80 days after sowing, and then decreased fairly rapidly during the period of vegetative growth, but changed little between anthesis and plant maturity.

In the female plants, also the highest fibre percentage was reached after 80 days, but this percentage was lower than in the male plants, although the intrinsic fibre yield at this stage was virtually the same for both. The period of rapid growth was about 30 days, in the male plants, ending before the peak of flowering, but lasted at least 40 days in the female plants, continuing to a less marked degree throughout fruit set and seed maturation. Thus the decrease in fibre percentage was more gradual and protracted in female than in the male plants. The most profitable time for harvesting the crop was at the end of male anthesis.

Hanin[154] investigated the effect of application of superphosphate on the fibre yields.

He found that on land treated with NK, superphosphate applied with seeds in the rows was about as effective as a 3-fold rate broad cast.

The highest fibre and seed yields were obtained from 15 kg. P_2O_5 per ha. applied in the rows.

Pamplona[254] experimented thirteen Korean, Italian and Japanese varieties for their fibre content. He also determined the relationships between the fibre contents at the ball-setting stage and at the maturity stage, the primary fibre content and the total fibre content. He found that the Italian varieties contained more fibre than the other varieties and there was a close correlation between the fibre contents at the ball-setting stage and the maturity stage, so that early selection is possible. Regression equations are given.

Anatomical studies showed that Italian varieties had wide bands of primary and secondary fibres with narrow bands of woody material, the revers was true of other varieties.

Stankovic[293] records development of a new methods for the mechanical extraction of fibres from hemp stalks.

He states that one new type of decorticating machine SC-32 has been developed and it increased the ratio between the extracted long and short fibres to 74.5 : 25.5%, while the standard types of machines decorted 60 : 40 percent.

14. Anatomy

Kundu[198, 199] investigated the development anatomy of *Cannabis* with special reference to fibre distribution. He was the first to record the fine structure of phloem fibres under different chemical treatments.

Herich[162, 163, 164] carried out histological investigations after subjecting the plants to gibberellic acid treatments. he found that the stems of female hemp plants raised from seeds treated with 5 ppm. G.A. on comparison with non-treated ones showed that they were thinner and the lower third portion of axis showed more strongly developed xylem and pith cavity, while a lower proportion of the cortex, the middle portion and the xylem poorly developed. There was an increase in phloem and parenchymatous tissues, while in the upper third there is decreased in xylem and the size of the pith cavity.

Heslop-Harrison[168] studied the effect of 2-thiouracil on cell differentiation and leaf morphogenesis in *Cannabis sativa*. he found that when it was supplied through the leaf at low dosage level, the pyrimidine analogue, 2-thiouracil, progressively arrests apical growth and organogenesis in young plants. During the treatment period, a generation of leaves arises in which cell differentiation is inhibited without a parallel reduction in laminal expansion. With the withdrawal of treatment, apical growth is resumed, but severe morphogenetic effects later become evident in leaves developing from primorida initiated during the treatment period or shortly afterwards and there is simultaneously a loss of apical dominance and of the control of phyllotaxis. Growth of a more normal pattern is, however, gradually restored at stem species, although local anomalies in the anatomy of the lamina recur throughout the life of the plant, and otherwise normal leaves continue to show sporadic flecks or streakings of abnormal pigmentation.

The latter phenomenon suggests that the analogue induces a persistent state of instability in some of the protoplastids of meristematic tissues.

Kalisevic and Porohnevic[187] investigated the effects of gibberellic acid on anatomical structures of *Cannabis* stems. They followed the following procedure:

Two drops of a 0.01% GA solution were applied daily to the tips of *Cannabis* plants grown in nutrient solution for 30 days, beginning one week after sowing. This treatment was found to increase the number of bast fibres visible in a cross section by about 37% and increased the length of the fibres by about 29%.

The diameter and wall thickness of the fibres were not significantly affected. The thickness of the xylem vessel walls was increased by about 30% by the GA treatment.

Metcalfe and Chalk[235] outlines the characteristic features of *Cannabis*.

Novak et al[249, 250] developed some anatomical criteria for separating *C. sativa Linn* var. *indica* from ordinary varieties.

Schilling[280] recorded some diagnostic characters of bast fibres from the study of various varieties of *Cannabis*.

Stant[291] found that treatment of plants of *Cannabis sativa* with GA induced highly significant increase in cell diameter and wall thickness of phloem fibres. This difference varied along the shoot and was maximal in the middle region, internodes 10-15. The ratio of cell-wall thickness to cell breadth was higher in treated plants. G.A. reduced the angle of orientation of the pits to the cell wall and also the pit frequency.

Pits in treated plants were longer and narrower in surface view.

Treggi[314, 315] observed in effect of sodium on the development of fibro-vascular bundles in *Cannabis*. He noticed that fibre quantity and quality were best in cultures with Na at 6% fairly good with Na at 12%.

The sand-cultures were supplied with cations K, Mg, Ca and Na, by means of dusarite, K and Mg. each forming 6% of cation total, Na forming 0, 3, 6, 12 or 18%, while Ca the remainder.

The lowest application had a slight beneficial effect and the highest none.

Zander[343] investigated the anatomy of *Cannabis sativa*.

15. Pests

Takalic[309] was one of those who suggested a biomethod for the control of stem borer on *Cannabis* in which he states that the release at the end of the June, when the *Cannabis* plants are 14 cm. high of 66, 000-100,000 eggs per ha. of *Trichogramma* considerably reduced the number of borers (*Pyrausta* (caterpillars. In one case the parasite reduced damage to 6.7-30% of that found on the control plants.

Manolache, Sandru and Romascu[222] records *Grapholitha delineata* Wall-(Lapidoptera-Tortricidae) as a pest on *Cannabis* crops.

16. Entomology

Goidanich, Athos[145] reviews the entomological fauna which attacks *Cannabis* (canapa) plants in Emilia. He records 102 species and varieties, their parasites and predators (81 species and varieties).

The species are divided into biocoenoses according to the part of the plant which they attack. The roots have been found infected by the larvae of the beetles *Psylliodes attenuata* Koch, *Melolontha melolantha* L., and *M. hippocastani* F.

The inside of the stem is destroyed by (1) *Pyrausta nubilialis* Hubn (parasites : *Phaeogenes nigridens* Wesm: *Pristomerus vulnerator* Panz, which has a pteromaline hyper-parasite, *Microgaster globatus* Nees, which has a ptermaline hyperparasite.

Eulophus sp: species of pteromalines; *Megaselia goidanichi* Schmitz; species of tachinid, with a pteromaline hyperparasite. Commensals : *Forficula aurcularia L; Tetramorium caepitum* L; *Elachiptera cornuta* Fall. (parasites : *Allotria minuta* Holm; *Loxotropa parva* Thoms); *Siphonella* nucis Perr; *Chyliza permixta* Rond; *Aseia elegantula* Zett; *Scaptomyza flaveola Meig*. (Parasites *Callitula elongata* Thoms; C. sp; and a species of pteromaline); *Ceutorrhynchus rapae* Gyll; *Mordellistema* sp. (parasite : sp. of ptermamline). Numerous Hemiptera, Homoptera and Auchenorhyncha. *Eulecanium* sp; and *Phorodon cannabis* spoils the textile properties of the fibres of the stem.

The stems of the juvenile plants are completely devoured by *Rhyacia ypsilon* Rott (Syn. *Qurotis suffusa v. pepoli* Bertol.); gryllus chinensis Web; and *G. desertus* Pall. The leaves are minced by *Phyto-myza atricornis* Meig. The (Parasites: *Dacnusa areolaris* Nees; *Closterocerus formosus* Westiv; *Derostenus* sp; *Pleurotropis* sp; etc.); and *Agromyza strigata*.

The stem is punctured by *Grapholitha compositella* F. The leaves are eaten by *Ematurga atomaria* L., and var. *Orientaria* stgr; (parasites : *Apanteles obscurus* Nees.): *Lycia hirtaria* Cl: species of geometrids (parasites: *Microplitis tuberculifera* Wesm; *Phylactor chlorophthalmus* Hal; *Anilastus ruficincuts* Grav; and *Litomastix truncatellus* Dalm.); *Cnephasia wahlbomiana* L. (parasites: *Trichomma enecator* Rossi; Elachertus sp.); *Bucculatrix ulmella* Zell; *Phytometra gamma* L; *Rhyacia ypsilon* Rott; *Barathra brassicae* L; *Lymantria dispar* L; Species of Lepidoptera. (parasites : *Nemeritis macrocentra* Grav; *N. convergens* Thoms; *Bassus laetatorius* F; and *Angitia cerophaga* Grav.); *Phaneroptera quadripunctata* Brunn; *Tettigonia contans* Fues; *ceutorrhynchus rapae* Gyll; *Apin ochropus; A. nigritarse; A. flavipes; A. apricans; A. aestivum; A. pisi; A. tenue; Sitnes lineatus* L; *S. sulcifrons* Thumb; *S. humeralis* Steph; *Psylliodes attenuata* Koch; and numerous other Colopetra and Lepidoptera. The leaves are punctured to obtain sap, by numerous Hemiptera and Homoptera.

The flowers are destroyed by *Calocoris norvequcus* Gemel; *ceutorrhynchus rapae* var *Sol; C. sulcicollis* Payk; *Sibinia pellucens* Scop; *Sitones lineatus; S. sulcifrons; S. himeralis; Psylliodes attenuata, Pyrrhia umbra* Hufn; (parasite : *Phytodietus* rufipes Holm.) The fruit, capsules are devoured by *barathra brassica* L. The fertility of the flowers in decreased or destroyed by the puncture of *Phorodon cannabis* Pass. (parasites : *Pachyneuron* sp; *Aphidius scabiosae* Marsh. (hyper parasitized by *Aphidencyrtus aphidivorus* Mayr.); *Aphidius* sp; *Blacus ruficornis* Nees; (Hyepr parasitized by *Bracon fulvipes* Nees and *B. variator* Nees.); *Spilomicrus minor* kieff; predators *Chrysopa perla* L. (parasitized by *Hemiteles aestivalis* Grav.) *Melanostoma mellinum* L; *Spihaerophoria scripta* L; (parasitized by *Homocidus tarsatorius* Panz); *Nabis rugosus* L; *N. ferus* L; *N. myrecoides* Costa (preyed upon by *Dinetus pictus* L.) and nuerous species and varieties of Coccinellidae).

Two species of ant which visit and sterilize Phorodon are : *Formica fusca* sp. *rufibarbis* F. and *Camponotus piceus* Leach.

Maximum damage to *Cannabis* is done by *Pyrausta nubilalis, Psyliodes attenuata, Phorodon cannabis, Ceutorrhynchus rapae, Calocoris norvequcus* and *Gryllus* species.

17. Virus-Bacteria

Phatak and Batra[258] noticed in vitro effects of apolenic antibiotic (pentaene 8) produced by *Streptomyces anandi* on SMV (Sann hemp mosiac) virus.

Goldanich and Ferri[146] found that a strain of *Pseudomonas canabina* was found as a pathogen causing bacteriosis, on *Cannabis* in Italy.

18. Fungi

Barloy[38] records that 120 types of *Cannabis* collected from different parts of the world, some Greek, Lebanese, Italia, (Carmagnola) and Romanian strains have proved to be least susceptible to broomrape (*Orobanche ramosa*).

Ferri[129] investigated the micro-flora of *Cannabis* seed. He found that species of fungi vary one hemp seeds from different sources. Furthermore, none of the seeds disinfectants used completely eradicated the fungi, but the best treatment was immersion from 5-10 minutes in 0.1% corrosive sublimate (mercuric chloride).

In ordinary soil seeds free from visible infection until the radicle had reached a length of 1-2mm. were not attacked by any of the fungi inoculated into the soil, but only by *Fusarium roseum*, which was present inside the seeds. Very few species attacked seeds in soil inoculated after sterilization, but several gained entry from vermiculite. *Alternative tenius* and Rhizopus nigricans were the only pathogenic fungi causing appreciable mortality in the open after seed treatment with corosive sublimate.

Further, he[131] studied the seed-transmitted disorders of Italian Hemps.

He found leaf crinkling, with chlorosis of the interveinal tissues, is transmitted by 40-50 percent of the seeds of affected hemp plants.

Although it cannot be transmitted by grafting or by sap injection, it is possibly a virus infection.

Deformity is a less common defect in which the plants are stunted and grow spirally, and the leaves droop. It is carried by 50-60 percent of the seeds of affected plants and is not transmitted by sap inoculation insect or grafting.

Chlorosis appears about midsummer and develops rapidly causing heavy losses in seed production; it is transmitted by 40-50% of the seeds of effected plants. Spotted chlorosis is characterized by male polygonal spots on the leaves, expanding and finally becoming confluent is in the other form of chlorosis, the defect is inherent in 30-40% of the seeds, Neither form of chlorosis is sap-transmitted. In general, the standard hemp varieties are more resistant than the new, high yielding types.

Ferri and Noviello[132] carried out investigations on the control of Sclerotium rolfsii on Italian hemp.

They found that in pot experiments the infection of *Cannabis* by *Sclerotium rolfsii* was almost completely prevented by presowing soil disinfection with 2 percent commercial formalin, where as 0.3% Ceresan, (Containing ethyl mercury chloride) was much less effective and 0.1% Amicine (a chinosol product) had no significant action. Of these three products in vitro only Ceresan failed to give 100 percent inhibition of sclerotial germination. Coltal at 0.35% (a 1:10:20 mixture of Chinosol, IMTD, and Zineb in an inert base) had a reasonably good curative action, but was surpassed by Brassicol at 0.2% (equal parts of PCNB and chalk).

In field experiments the results were modified by the nature of the soil, a heavy clay with deep cracks favouring the activity of the fungus. Soil disinfection with formalin was the only significant preventive treatment, but was less effective against natural than against artificial infection. The curative action of Brassicol was significant, but not outstanding and that of Coltal was practically nil.

Ljusinskij[214] experimented with 160 Russian and foreign hemp varieties over 2 years, for resistance to broomrape (*Orobanche ramosa*) and first and second generation of hemp flea beetle (*Psylliodes attenuata*). Of the greatest interest were two Hungarian varieties V-7 and Kompolti–V-7 L, which were resistant to both broomrape and the first generation of flea beetles.

He found that there exists a relationship between the origin and morphological characters on the one hand, and resistance to both parasites on the other.

19. Diseases

Darloy and Pelhate[38] observed that *Cannabis* fibre yields are practically unaffected by broomrape (*Phelipea, (orobanche) ramosa*) if less than 1 in 40 of the plants become hosts, but if the proportion, rises to 1 in 5-6, a 30 percent yield reduction may be expected. When infestation is still heavier, the only means of avoiding total crop failure is the very early harvesting.

Good control has been achieved by spraying the newly emerged broomrape inflorescences with hormone herbicides, carefully avoiding the *Cannabis* foliage. Susceptibility to the parasite is lower in dioecious than in monoecious varieties.

Certain Russian and Romanian varieties, claimed to be immune, have been attacked in Anjou.

Early and liberal application of N to the crop reduces the injury due to broomrape. The fly-*Phytomyza orobanchiae* destroys broom rape seeds and, if introduced sufficiently early, would probably be a useful supplementary controlling factor.

the fungus *Fusarium orobanchae* has been successfully used in Russia to destroy broomrape.

Dodder (*Cuscuta monogyna*) causes little damage to *Cannabis* crops, but makes harvesting difficult, its control necessitates the thorough screening of *Cannabis* seed, especially that imported from Syria and the Lebanon. This seed is also a source of leaf spot (*Septoria cannabina*) infection.

Alternaria porri f. *solani* is a late season leaf pathogen against which fungicidal treatments would be uneconomic except when prolonged drought favours heavy infection.

Mildew (*Pseudoperonospora (Peronospora) cannabina*) merits control only on the susceptible Cannabis varieties imported from Iran and the Lebanon.

Didymella arcuata (Ascohyta cannabina) hitherto regarded as a leaf infection, appears only on the stems of *Cannabis* in Anjou.

Botrytis infestans often associated with *B. cinerea* severely damages the stems and inflorescences.

Curative measures are ineffective, but seed disinfection is to be tested. Control of the late season stem pathogen *Dendrophoma marconii (Botryosphaeria marconii)* is uneconomic.

Fusarum oxysporum and *F. solani* are most harmful to crops on light, alluvial soils, that are continually changing in water content.

Plants already attacked by broomrape are highly susceptible. The only method of control appears to be crop rotation.

20. Insecticides

Manninger, Boscsa and Klement[221] studied the phytotoxic effects of contact insecticides on *Cannabis*.

They found that bacterial and mycological tests were negative in tumescences observed on the main roots of Cannabis at Kompolt in 1954 and these were ascribed to the phytotoxic action of BHC dustings. In trials in 1955 and 1956, BHC preparations either proved lethal or produced similar symptoms, whereas DDT formulations were innocuous. These findings were confirmed in 1957. A high soil moisture content enhanced phytotoxicity. On sandy soils even low rates of BHC were apt to cause injury.

21. Narcotics Produced

Narcotic drugs obtained from *Cannabis indica* are Bhang (Hashish, Marihuana), Ganja and Charas.

The methods of preparation and types of plants used for extracting the drugs vary.

In India, the pistillate plants are pruned in order to produce flowering branches which are then collected, allowed to wilt and pressed by treading them under the feet into compact flattened masses. The drug thus produced is exported from Bombay and is known in London market as "Guaza" or "Ganja".

In the East Bengal districts, the gathered flowering tops are rolled under the feet of men who support themselves by bamboo poles and thus produce round masses of drug. This variety is termed as Bengal "Ganja" and is said to be physiologically more active, it is rarely sent to England, but smuggled out of India. It comes from plants with larger leaves and dried young twigs, and forms and `Bhang' which is also consumed in India.

There is still another method of extracting the drug. It is not beat the plant by cloths to which resin adheres; a greenish-brown soft mass is thus obtained which is freed from plant debris by warming and pressing through cloth. This product is termed as 'Charas' and like 'Ganja' is smoked by Indians and Eastern races with the object of producing an agreeable form of intoxication. Commercial products of this drug usually occur as flattened, compressed, rough masses of dull green colour, which are resinous to touch. The pieces vary in length from 5 to 30 cm. consisting of a straight stem with ascending branches bearing numerous curved hairs and stalked glands, the latter secreting a viscid adhesive resin.

Chemical Constituents

A number of pure cannabinoids have been isolated from *Cannabis*. The most important cannabinoids which produce ataxia in the dog and psychotomimetic effects in man are : Δ^{1-} transtetrahydrocannabinol and Δ^{16-} transtetrahydrocannabinol. Tetrahydrocannabinol carboxylic acid has yet to be biologically evaluated.

Indian *Cannabis* contains a resin which is said to be responsible for narcotic action. This can be separated as a soft brown substance-Cannabinone, from which by distillation under reduced pressure a viscous resin can be separated. This melts to an oily liquid when warmed, and forms Cannabinol. On exposure to air it rapidly loses its activity. It takes an year for deterioration. Each plant produces 15-20% total resin. In addition to cannabinone the drug contains traces of the base choline and a small amount of volatile oil.

The ash (Mineral mater) varies between 15-18%, while alcohol extract shows 18-20 percent. The material extracted by alcohol loses cannabinol due to oxidation.

Identification of Indian Cannabis

Powdered specimens can be identified as follows: 0.1 gm. of powdered sample is macerated for 3 minutes with 5 ml of petroleum ether and the liquid filtered.

To 1 ml. of the filtrate, 2 ml. of a 15% solution of hydrogen chloride in absolute alcohol is added.

A red colouration appears at the junction of the two immiscible liquids if positive, and on shaking the upper layer becomes colourless while the liquid beneath is orange-pink in colour. It disappears on addition of 1 ml. of water. (cf. Allport[18]).

There are several methods that can be used for the detection of *Cannabis* in cigarettes, or when mixed with other plant materials.

Chemical Tests

(i) *Beam test* : This simply involves extraction of the suspected samples with petroleum ether, evaporation of the solvent and the addition of a few drops of alcoholic potassium hydroxide to the residue. The production of a violet colour is taken as an evidence that the sample contains *Cannabis*. The reaction is a test for the presence of the inactive cannabidiol, cannabidiolic acid and other constituents, but do not give positive test, including the tetrahydrocannabinols, Several other plants may give false-positive reactions to this test. It is claimed that these can be eliminated for the most part by shaking the violet colour reaction mixture of a positive test with chloroform and allowing the chloroform and water layers to separate. If the reaction is a false-positive one, the violet colour will not migrate into the chloroform layer[232].

(ii) *Ghmravy test* : This involves the use of dimethylamino benzaldehyde and sulfuric acid.

(iii) *Duquenois-Negm test* : This involves vanillin, acetaldehyde and ethanol, the modified Duquenois-Negm test, which involves hydrochloric acid followed by extraction with chloroform.

(iv) *Fast blue salt test* : This involves the fast salt B reagent which gives various colours with the phenolic cannabinoids.

(v) *The garlic test* : This involves the use of hydrogen peroxide and sulfuric acid.

(vi) *Thin-layer chromatography*: In this petroleum ether extract from a suspected Cannabis containing sample is subjected to rapid simple inexpensive and accurate assessment of the specific cannabinoid content of the sample, both from a qualitative as well as from a semi-quantitative point of view. Rapid development of the sample on Kieselgel G. plates is followed, impregnated with N, N-di-methylformamide and using cyclohexane as the eluent, the various cannabinoids can be separated into well-defined spots. Each chromatogram is treated with fast blue salt B reagent, resulting in the production of several colours for the separated components. Tetrahydrocannabinol forms a scarlet colour, cannabinol shows violet, cannabidiol and cannabidiol carboxylic acid are orange, cannabichromene is brownish-violet and cannabicyclol is brick red. The Rf values of the separated components offer additional evidence for their identification. (Grlic, L-Bull. Narcotics, 16(4), 29 (1964).

(vii) *Gas chromatography*: The identification of *Cannabis* samples by means of gas chromatography is unique by itself. The instrument is expensive, the technique requires some degree of skill for its operation and maintenance. Reference samples are a necessity.

Microscopic Tests

Since plants bear numerous hairs of two types, these are useful in the identification.

(i) Hairs with cystolith containing a crystal of calcium carbonate in the basal portion of hair. If a mineral acid is added to am icroscopic preparation of the suspective samples of *Cannabis*, the calcium carbon crystal in the basal portion of the hair decomposes with effervescence (carbon dioxide).

(ii) There are also present characteristic resin-producing multicellular grandular hairs.

The presence of these two types of plant hairs in a sample can be safely regarded as the presence of *Cannabis*.

Biological evaluation

The most common method for detecting *Cannabis* activity is to administer the sample to a dog and observe for signs of ataxia.

Types of Cannabis

Bhang, Siddhi, Sabji or Patti are different names applied to the same type of product. It consists mostly of specially dried leaves and flowering shoots of both the male and female *Cannabis* plant. At times it may show admixture of seeds. 'Bhang' is obtained from plants growing wild in Bihar, Bengal, Assam, U.P. and Punjab.

Bhang is Prepared from plants cut, alternately exposed to sun and dew, and when dry the leaves are pressed and stored in earthen-ware vessels. The usual time for gathering the leaves is May to June in the plains, and June to July in the hills.

It is consumed in the form of sweet meats or in a form of pounded leaves with species and swallowed in the form of a bolus.

Ganja consists of dried flowering and fruiting tops of the female plant from which no resin has been removed. The "Flat" (Bombay ganja) which is exported to the United kingdom, occurs in agglutinated flattened masses of dull green or greenish brown colour. The resin is no longer sticky, but hard and brittle; the odour which is very marked in the fresh drug, is faint.

The drug has a slightly bitter taste.

There are two types of ganja namely (i) Flat or 'Bombay ganja' and (ii) 'Round' or 'Bengal ganja'. It is prepared by rolling the withered tops into small rounded or sausage shaped masses between the hands. The broken fragments and powder of 'flat' and 'round' ganja constitute the 'Chur-Ganja' or 'Rora'.

Ganja of good quality yields '5-25% resin on extraction with carbon tetrachloride; the ash content does not exceed 15%.

Cannabis B.P.C. contains about 10% fruits, large foliage leaves and stems over 3mm. diameter, and not more than 2% foreign organic matter. It shows acid insoluble ash 5%; matter soluble in alcohol after drying at 100°, not less than 10%.

Ganja is used mostly for smoking in a pipe (Chilam) after mixing with a little water and tobacco.

Charas : consists of the resinous exudation collected from the leaves of Cannabis plant. It is imported from 'Yarkand' (Central Asia) as plants growing in that area are said to produce highest yield of good quality resin.

'Charas' is dark-green when fresh and becomes brown on

exposure. The resin content of good quality charas is about 40% (range 35-35%), but the potency of the drug is not recognised by its resin contents. Long storage and contact with air deteriorates the potency of the drug.

22. Pharmacognosy

Farnsworth[126, 127] has outlined in details the pharmacognostic characteristics of *Cannabis sativa*.

23. Mode of consumption

In India 'Bhang' is either taken as a beverage, or swallowed as confection or chewed; on the other hand 'ganja' and 'Charas' are smoked.

(i) *Beverages* : In Bengal it is known as Siddhi, in United Provinces as Bhang, in Western peninsular as Ghota, in Rajasthan as 'dudhi', while in Southern India as 'Ram rasain'. By whatever vernacular name it is known, the beverage is used by the poorer castes who drink the pounded leaves with black pepper and sugar. Not infrequently it is enriched by additions of almonds, curds, cucumber seeds, rose petals, cloves, cardamom and musk. Pistachio nuts, extracts from various herbs and also added.

(ii) Confections: In United Provinces, Bihar, and Bengal 'bhang' preparations are quite well known. They prepare 'Majum'–a fried leaves of *Cannabis* mixed with sugar and condensed milk, 'Halwa'–a jaggery syrup added with wheat flour and fats, 'Curry' leaves in combination with ordinary vegetable curry.

Common Admixtures

Datura seeds (*Datura innoxia*) are commonly used by addicts to increase narcotic effect of *Cannabis*. Less frequently juice of *Calotropis gigantea*, (since it is a common weed), opium, arsenic and sometimes strychnine, are added. Not infrequently the Bhang decoction is "steeped" with a red hot copper coin, to make it more potent.

A very dangerous decoction called 'madra' is prepared with seeds of *datura*, Opium, *Cannabis* and alcohol and in certain parts of Baluchistan.

Cannabis drugs have been used to induce a state of

intoxication during frequent encounters with Muslim invaders in old days in India. Bhang was also used to banish fear and nervousness. Robbers and dacoits now take these drugs to indulge in cruel acts during intoxication.

24. Addiction

The use of Cannabis for intoxication originated from Asia, from where it has spread to the eastern and southern coasts of Africa and to certain parts of the United States.

Since of its wide use, several varieties and the forms of this plant has been developed in various countries, the nomenclature of the plant therefore, differs.

In India, bhang, ganja and charas are obtained from *Cannabis* and are used as *narcotics*.

The resin separated from *Cannabis* is known as hashish in the Middle East. Dried leaftops and tender parts are smoked and chequed in Arabia, Egypt, Turkey and North African countries.

Cannabis was introduced into South Africa from the East by sailors going around the Cape. The plant is known as 'dagga' and is mainly used by Bantu tribes.

In Brazil, *Cannabis* is known as Maconha but is also commonly known by other names like 'diamba', 'fumo de Angola', Pango, liamba, dirijo, birra, elva, and finninha. In Central America and in Mexico it is known as 'marihuana' or 'Rosa Maria' D. Juanita' Maconha (*Cannabis*) is smoked through cigarettes or special pipes known in Brazil as 'Maricas'.

Maconha consists of dried leaves, flowering stalks and fruits of *Cannabis*. They are called by different depending upon the quantity it contains, viz. A 2.5 g portion is known as 'Morrao' while 1.7 g as 'Baseado' a nd 1.0 g. part as 'fininho'.

Marihuana is known to Mexican aborigines who used it during their religious ceremonies. It was introduced in New Orleans as early as 1910, probably by seasonal Mexican labourers in the United States. Sailors too were found to be engaged in business of this narcotic. Peddlers seem to be mostly Mexicans, Italians, Spanish-Americans, who were drifter from the ships. New Orleans appears to be a distribution centre, from where *Cannabis* is shipped to Mississippi into all river ports. The drug seems to have reached as far north as Cleveland, Ohio. Smoking of Marihuana has become a problem since it has found its way even among school children. Marihuana cigarettes go under the name of 'Mootas'.

Another country where *Cannabis* is smoked is *Tibet*. It is known by the name of 'Momea' or 'Mimea'—a *Cannabis* preparation said to be made with human fat(!)

Furthermore, its wide-spread use as an intoxicant and in cultic use of psychotomimetics justifies classifying *Cannabis* in a position between psychotomimetics and narcotics.

25. Newer chemical investigations

Aramaki Hanichiro et al[29] developed a new detection method for various Marihuana constituents which is of a practical use in identification of *Cannabis*. They found that Cannabidiol, tetrahydrocannabinol, and cannabinol in marihuana samples can be effectively detected in the smoke condensate and in the resin by thin-layer chromatography with C_6H_6-hexane-Et_2NH (25:10:1) and diazotized benzidine as a developer and by gas chromatography with 1.5% S.E. 30 on Chromosorb W at 220°. This identification was not interfered with by the presence of tobacco or *Humulus lupulus* akin to *Cannabis sastiva*. In the smoking experiment, 50 percent vaporized in the smoke and half of the vapour was absorbed on the cigarette filters.

Agurell Stig-Nissson et al[11] experimented with the excretion of *Cannabis* compounds in the urine. They found that after i.p. injection of a *Cannabis* extract in olive oil (50 mg/kg body weight) in rats, a 24 hour urine collection was extracted with petroleum ether and the extract purified by thin-layer chromatography on silica gel. They found that compounds were not excreted in the urine unchanged, less than 0.003% of the administered extract was excreted free or conjugated with glucuronic acid. A^3H-labelled extract was injected i.p. into rats and urine and faeces were collected until no more activity could be detected. Excretion was slow and 70-80% of the excreted material was found in the faeces and 10 to 20% in the urine.

Betts and Holoway[45] outline quite an other reliable method of chromatographic identification of Cannabis. This could be achieved by using thin-layer chromatography together with gas chromatography. This eliminates false positive reactions which adulterants of labiate herbs record with one or other of the chromatographic methods if used alone. Tops and resin have been examined. The classic *Cannabis* colour reactions have been used as sprays for thin-layer chromatography. During gas chromatography a 2% silicone elastomer on a silianized support was used, and cannabinols were run as their trimethylsilyl ethers.

Bozner[55] evolved another method by use of paper chromatography for distinguishing different *Cannabis* varieties by means of acid and alkaline hydrolysates and alcohol extracts from young *Cannabis* plants. He found that the position, size and intensity of the spots produced on the chromatograms of these extracts by simple sugars were used to identify hemp varieties and establish affinities between them.

Cahn[71, 72, 73] investigated the resin and pointed out the constitution of cannabinol.

Crombie, and Ponsford[101] synthesized hashish cannabinoids by terpenic cyclization. They found that when a mixture of olivetol I more citral and 1 mole pyridine is heated 7 hours at 110% gives 15% cannabichromene, 26 percent citrylidene cannabis, 1% cannabicyclol (cannabipinol-m. 146°), 3% isocannabichromene, 3% isocannabicyclol, 6% bischromene and 1.5% biscyclobutance (m. 122-3°).

Caddy and Fish[70] evolved a screening technique for Indian *Cannabis* by two thin-layer chromatography, whereby several samples can be screened simultaneously for major cannabinolic compounds in about an hour's time.

Davis, Farmilo and Osadchuk[108] outline a method of identification and determination of different constituents by gas and paper chromatography. In this method 4 active principles (Cannabinols) in the leaves and in the flowers could be identified. Further-more, samples from different countries show characteristic variation in the proportions of the 4 compounds which are correlated with the differences in the climatic conditions.

Farmilo and Davis[125] evolved a new method for analysis of resin of *Cannabis indica* by means of paper and gas-chromtography.

Fujita Mituti et al[135] examined the narcotic and its related compounds, both in crude drugs and in plant organs (Marihuana, Ganja and charas) by gas liquid chromatography and thin-layer chromatography.Δ^9-Tetrahydro-cannabinol was found in the female inflorescence both in wild and cultivated species of *Cannabis sativa* Linn. independent of their condition. The cannabis components were detected in petroleum ether extract obtained from each organ of the Japanese *Cannabis*-Manami-Oshihara No.1, at the time of fructification. Cannabidiol is a main component in the first green leaves after the time of germination of Minami-Oshihara species. Results by gas liquid chromatography show that these components were not find in the oily part of the disk shaped glandular hair collected using a micromanipulator technique, but they were detected in the resin canal and the secretory cells of the glandular hair which seem to have resin content. The phenolic components of *Cannabis* were not found in ash obtained from Minami-Oshihara variety of *Cannabis*, while in Ganja-smoke (Indian) large amount of unchanged cannabi-diol, cannabinol, cannabigerol and Δ^9-tetrahydro-cannabinol were found in the filter through which the smoke passed.

Gaoni and Mechoulam[137] isolated tetrahydrocannabinol from female flowering tops of *Cannabis sativa*.

Gantra et al[139] investigated the seizure samples of Cannabis indica and subjected them for critical identification. They could separate each sample by comparative microscopic examination, T.L. chromatography and corneal areflexia tests.

Herich and Priechardny[159] noticed the variations found in the sugar content and reducing capacity of tissues of the root and aerial parts of male, female and monoecious *Cannabis* plants. Further they studied the differences in N.P. and K. contents in relation to sex differentiation.

Kane, Razdan, and Ray[188] investigation different constituents of hashish and found that on heating equimolar amounts of olivetol, citral and pyridine a complex product mixture in which they were able to identify dl–Δ^1 (6)-3-4-transtetrahydrocannabinol, $\Delta^{4(8)}$-isotetrahydrocannabinol, 3, 3a, 4, 5–tetrahydro-2, 5, 5-trimethyl–8–pentyl-2, 4 ethano 2H-pyrano (4, 3, 2,-de) (1), benzopyran, cannabicyclol, cannabichromene, dl–Δ^1–3, 4–cis–tetrahydrocannabinol and dl–Δ^1–3, 4trans-tetrahydrocannabinol.

Kingston and Kirk[192] developed a method of separation of components of marijuana by gas-liquid chromatography. They could obtain date on 6 fractions from *C. Sativa* resin.

Korte and Sieper[195] were able to determine cannabidiol, tetrahydrocannabinol and cannabinol spectrometrically after separation by thin-layer chromatography and the formation of azp-derivatives. They suggest that this method can be useful for determination of crude extract of *Cannabis* and its varieties.

Further they[194] were able to separate from synthetic (tetrahydrocannabinols) by chromatographic and counter current distribution methods, two crystalline isomers.

Martin, Smith and Farmilo[219] found that gas chromatograms taken of fresh oil from *Cannabis sativa* showed a constant pattern of 14 peaks, which gives a reliable characterization for forensic purposes. Dried *Cannabis* charas and hashis could also be identified with this technique.

Mechoulam, Ben-Zvi, and Gaoni[232] revealed the nature of the Beam test. According to them, the purple colour produced by treatment of Cannabidiol with 5% ethanolic KOH (Beam test) is due to the anions of the hydroxyquinone and its dimer. The latter two are formed from cannabidiol by air oxidation during the reaction. The diquinone III is reduced in the mass spectrometer to M++4 species (probably the dihydroquinone).

Further they[233] noticed that when they treated Δ^{1}- 3, 4-transtetrahydrocannabinol (Δ^{1}- 3, 4–trans-THC) with chloranil in C_6H_6 it gave cannabinol, while under identical conditions Δ^{1} (6)-THC, Δ^{1}- 3, 4–cis–THC, cannabidiol and 5–hydroxy–2–methyl–7. Pentyl–2– (4-emthyl–3–pentenyl) chroman were recovered unchanged, indicating that chloranil dehydration involved a stereo-electronic factor. Chloranil dehydrogenation of cannabigerol gave 45% dl-cannabichromene, and the former 15%.

Mechoulam[231] describes the structure of cannabidiol based on its nuclear magnetic resonance spectrum.

Nigam[247] investigated the essential oil obtained by hydro-distillation of freshly harvested Indian *Cannabis sativa* and found that it contained X-pinene, comphene, B-pinene, X-terpinene, B-phellandrene, X-terpinene-linalool, trans-linalool oxide, sabinene hydrate, X-bergamotene, terpinene–4–ol, B-farnesene, X-terpineol, X-selinene, cururmene and caryophyllene oxide. The presence of trace amounts of 2 alcohols and of an –X-B–Unsaturated ketone were recorded by gas chromatographic and spectral analysis.

Novak, Haznagy and szendrei[251] found that Beam-chloride values and spectro-photometric curves were suitable for distinguishing Indian and Hungarian *Cannabis*. Furthermore, chemical and spectrophotometric studies confirmed that Hungarian varieties of *Cannabis* were devoid of narcotics.

St. Angelo et al[21, 22] were also able to isolate edestin from aleurone grains of *Cannabis sativa*. Aleurone grains, protein bodies, were isolated by employing a density gradient of carbon tetrachloride an d refined cotton-seed oil. Electron microscopic monitoring of a cross-section of aleurone grain showed them to be composed of 3 different components (i) large crystalloid substructures (ii) globoids, and (iii) other minor constituents. All are enveloped by a membrane. The crystalloids were extracted from the isolated aleurone grains by repeated washings with solutions of sodium chloride and sodium dedecyl sulfate, sedimentation co-efficient and electrophoretic analysis of solutions of crystalloids indicated that the crystalloids were composed of pure edestin and, therefore, established edestin as an aleurin. Further monitoring of the crystalloids by elections microscopy suggested that they have a pebby surface and are composed of repeating polygonal shaped units, even down to 80A° level.

Czechoslavia Medical Faculty[96] has outlined a comprehensive method of the analysis of Indian *cannabis* using thin-layer chromatography. It was found that the best results were achieved on the unimpregnated thin layers Kieselgel G. Merck if a mixture of benzene and ethyl alcohol in the ratio of 95:5 was used as the developing phase. These compounds proved to be most convenient for the detection of isolated strains, 2.6 of dibromguinonchlorimide Merck, twice diazotized benzidine or Echthlausalz B. merck, respectively. The Comparative standards of chromatographically pure isolated substances of cannabidiole acid, cannabidiole and tetraphydrocannabinole were used for the identification. A probative chemical analysis was carried out to establish the weight quotients of the extractive material together with the weight relations of the substances of the acidic or phenolic character including the chromatographic isolation of the individual chemically isolated fractions from the sample of standard hashish.

Yutaka[342] tested the seeds and seedlings for the presence and activity of amylase, mattase, pepsin, trypsin, erepsin, urease, catalase and nuclease; It was in very small amounts in *Cannabis sativa*, but other enzymes were also present. Lipase was slightly active in *Cannabis*.

26. Toxicity

Bromberg[63, 64] investigated the *Cannabis* intoxication. Lopez-Merino[212] made clinical examination of occupation disease found in hemp workers. It was daily and weekly spirographic tests, the possible factors which influence bronchostenotic effect through inhalation of hemp-dust, and they analysed the severity of emphysema and fibrosis which develops in the final stage of the disease.

27. Reaction of Drug on Man

Clark and Nakashima[93] administered *Cannabis* (Marihuana) to volunteer subjects in an attempt to determine its effects and behavioural toxicity. Dosage ranged from 12.5 mg. to 30 mg. A mild 'high' was produced in all subjects when given a 30 mg. dose. Drug effects were evident in one hour, and lasted upto 8 Hours. A series of physical and physiological tests were administered to the subjects. A number of performance tests were not effected by the drug. However, complex reaction time, digit code, memory tasks were impaired. There were numerous individual differences in test results and in the drug effects. The study pointed to 'Marihuana' unpredictable effects. They can vary with different individual and on the same individual at different times and circumstances.

Baker and Lucas[35] found that in 1966 psychiatric hospitals were asked to include the name of the drug concerned on a mental health index card, when drug despondency was recorded as th e cause of admission. In that year 82 cases of *Cannabis* addiction were reported, 79 case papers were obtained for a review of the role played by *Cannabis* in leading to admissions. The cases were allocated to the following groups: (i) toxic confusional states leading to admission - 8 cases. (iii) Other physical or psychiatric symptoms leading to admission-13 cases. (iv) *Cannabis* addiction as "a way life" leading to social deterioration and eventual admission 20 cases, and (v) insufficient evidence or inadequate records for a decision to be reached–29 cases.

Carakushansky, New and Gardner[77] reports a case of an infant with a terminal transverse deficit of portions of fingers of the left hand and syndactyly of the right hand with shortened fingers, whose mother is believed to have been exposed to lysergide and *Cannabis* during pregnancy.

Gtossmann[150] records the adverse reaction with *Cannabis* products. Six patients with emotional disorders associated with the use of ganja, bhang and hashis products prepared by Westerners in India from *Cannabis sativar* var. Indica are reported.

Graff[148] narrates the experiences and effects of *Cannabis* (Marihuana) and scopolamine 'High' on a nineteen year old female. She experienced an acute psychotic reaction after smoking *Cannabis* (Marihuana) soaked in scopolamine. Thirty minutes after smoking the mixture the subject became agitated, combative and developed delusions unlike any experienced with marihuana alone. The patient developed a feeling of 'going carzy' her girl friend appeared to her to be darker in colour, voices sounded like the ringing of a telephone, time and space perceptions were altered. A portion of the intoxication period was spent clinging to a bed trying not to fall off. The psychotic state began to reside in 12 hour, however, hallucinations occurred periodically for 24 hours. There was no residual psychotic effect. The possibility of a marihuana-scopolamine toxicity activating the latent psychosis does exist especially in the population most interested in taking drugs for pleasure.

Kales et al[185] in their investigations on drug dependency, stimulants and depressants state that *Cannabis* (Marihuana) may change time sense and visual and auditory perceptions; chronic use frequently indicates underlying psychologic disturbances needing psychotherapy.

Myers and Caldwell[244] investigated the effects of Marihuana (*Cannabis*) on auditory and visual sensations. They carried out tests to determine the effects of inhalation of crude *Cannabis* (Marihuana) on (i) alterations in auditory threshold; (ii) ability to discriminate between paired tones of fixed frequency and varying amplitude; (iii) ability to discriminate between paired tones of fixed amplitude and varying frequency; (iv) ability to match a light of variable illuminance to a standard light of fixed illuminance. In this study the control group smoked 300 mg. alfalfa cigarettes, and the experimental group smoked cigarettes containing 300 mg. of crude *Cannabis* (Marhuana) 1.3% delta-tetrahydrocannabinol content). None of the subjects had Marihuana before. The data failed to reveal significant differences in performance between the two groups. In studies with a college population which had previously smoked Marihuana, each subject was allowed to smoke to a 'biological end point' or "high". Generally this required 350-400 mg. of Marihuana. The subjects reporting a "high" failed to demonstrate objective changes other than those observed in the initial group.

28. Pharmacology

Aguas da Silva et al[10] studied cross-tolerance in rats among (–)-Δ^9-trans-tetrahy-drocannabinol (Δ^9-THC), *Cannabis* extract, mescaline, and lysergic acid diethylamide (LSD-25). They found *Cannabis* extracts were sensitive to mescaline sulfate and LSD–25 and vice-versa. In spite of the similarity of clinical symptoms produced in man by these drugs, the psychotomimetic effects of (–)-Δ^9-trans-tetrahydrocannabinol are probably produced by mechanisms different from those producing the effects of mescaline sulphate and LSD–25.

Burger[66] reports that cannabis resin and synthetic tetrahydrocannabinol shows a strong hypothermic effects in rats.

He states it is still undecided whether (Bhang, hashish, Marihuana) is primarily a centra stimulant or depressant or both. The characteristic physiological changes seen in man are increase in pulse rate, a slight rise in blood pressure, tremor, ataxia, veritgo, hyper roflexia, increased sensitivity to touch and pupillary dilation. A marked increase in appetite.

Goodman and Gilman[147] and Miras[237] investigated the pharmacological activity of tetrahydrocannabinol together with other derivatives of cannabinol, constituting the characteristic constituents of *Cannabis*. The active toxicity (LD) of tetrahydrocannabinol of natural source and also of cannabinol and cannabidiol, is over 10 g./kg. orally in mice and between 100 and 230 mg/kg. intravenously in mice, rabbits, and dogs. Distribution studies with 14–labelled tetrahydrocannabinol showed that 1Ū hours after intraperitioneal application in rats most of the activity is contained in the liver. Brain also recorded a measurable amount of radioactivity. Ataxia potency in animals seems to have parallel physic potency in man. Miras[237] noticed that people treated with *Cannabis* feel cold in their extremities.

Garriott, et al[141] screened eight compounds related to cannabinol or tetrahydrocannabinol. Acute toxicities are found. Prolongation of hexobarbital sleeping time, depression of normal activity in mice, and depression of arterial blood pressure in anesthetized dogs were characteristic actions. Two compounds decreased the length of electro shock-induced convulsions.

Valle, Lapa, Basrros and Gluace[318] carried out a comparative *bioassy* of male and female *Cannabis* crude resins, using abolition of the rabbit blink reflex. They found that *cannabis* preparations exhibited the same degree of activity. Vincent and chapple[320] records the evidence of liver damage to be rare in patients whose abuse was confined to the use of amphetamines, barbiturates or *Cannabis*. It is suggested that while some cases of jaundice in narcotic addicts are viral origin, transient liver damage is more often the results of either a direct hepatotoxic effect of heroin and cocaine used, pyrogens, or other contaminants injected unwittingly or to sub-clinical bacteremias due to the use of septic materials.

Rousinov and Athanasova-Shopova[274] records *Cannabis sativa* used for its *anticonsulive* activity in popular medicine in Bulgaria.

29. Psychiatry

Abelson[1] points out the evaluation of the consequences leading to the popularity of the usage of *Cannabis* (marihuana).

Keeler[190] investigated the adverse reactions of *Cannabis* (marihuana). He found in case reports stages of panic, gross confusion, depersonalization, depression, and paranoia following the use of marihuana in a student population. These reports of adverse reaction are interpreted in the light of the expected reaction to the drug and the nature of the populations studied.

Murphy [242] in his psychiatric review of *Cannabis* habit states that there is still much to be learnt about the effect of *Cannabis* on human mind. It seems probable that it has a highly complex influence, dependent on personality and culture as well as on the drug itself. Furthermore, there is still a need for a properly designed study into the frequency of symptoms at different levels of consumption. The medical reputation which *Cannabis* has in folk-medicine appears to have some justification since, although erratic in action, it possesses a number of valuable properties.

30. Allergy

Bouhuys et al[56] observed byssinosis in *Cannabis* workers. They found byssinosis, chronic cough and other chronic respiratory symptoms prevalent among workers exposed to dust of raw biologically retted, soft hemp. Within this group non-reactors and reactors could be distinguished by the absence or presence of a decrease of forced expiratory volume (FEV_1) during dust exposure on Mondays. The questionnaire interview under-estimated the extent of the worker's symptoms. Urinary excretion of a major histamine metabolite (1, 4-methylimidazolacetic acid; Me IAA) was higher on Mondays than on Wednesdays in those reactors whose FEV_1 decreased on Mondays but not an Wednesdays. Bronchocontrictive response to *Cannabis* dust exposure on Mondays is a result of the release of histamine in the lungs. A deleterious effect of long term hemp dust exposure upon pulmonary function is highly probable FEV_1 (before dust exposure, adjusted for age and height) was significantly lower among the *Cannabis* workers than among a control group (farm workers), although the latter smoked more and significantly lower among those with byssinosis grade 1 and 2, than among those without, or with mild symptoms of disease, 9 out of 20 retired *Cannabis*workers had an FEV_1 of Ū the expected value or less. Among the active workers[1] abnormally low values of FEV_1 (before dust exposure) were only found in reactors and not in non-reactors. Irreversible pulmonary function changes develop primarily in those individuals who are sensitive to be acute broncho-contrictive effect of dust.

Jimenez-Diaz et al[184] noticed occurrence of Asthma and fibrosis in two patients working with *Cannabis* and mattweed.

31. Anti-biotic Activity—Antibacterial

Ferency Gracza and Jakobey[133] were able to produce antibacterial preparation from the extracts of raisins organs of *Cannabis*.

Rabinovic, Ajzenman and Zelepuha[262] investigated the anti-microbial substances from wild Ukraine *Cannabis* (*C. ruderalis*). They found that dry leaves and tops of *C. ruderalis* yield 0.1% of essential oil (1: 50,000 to 1 : 100,000 activity), 0.002% of alkaloid (activity upto 1; 40,000) and 0.5% of a complex acids. The latter constitute the anti-bacterial compounds in wild hemps.

Radosevic, Kupinic and Grlic[263] found that increasing ripeness of resins of *Cannabis* was accompanied by the conversion of the anti-bacterial agent (cannabidiolic acid) to hashish-active constituents (tetrahydrocannabinols) with a consequent decrease in antibiotic activity. Antibiotic principles were present in plants of unfavourable climates, while hashish active constituents were present in species of warmer regions.

Martinec and Felklova[217, 218] noticed that the activity of Cannabis sativa varies quantitatively but not qualitatively according to the stage of development of the plant. Only the leaves and inflorescences are active, the root and stem being inactive. The maximum inhibitory effects of leaf extracts generally occurred in August and of inflorescences in September. Later in the season, there was a marked decline in activity. It was found that phosphorus fertilizer promoted the anti-bacterial activity of the leaves and especially the inflorescences.

32. International Control

Legal possession and laws on Marihuana has been outlined in Canadian Medical Association Journal in 1967. After World War II a Committee on Narcotic Drugs of the "Economic and Social Council" was constituted under the United Nations Organization. The Committee adopted an agreement known as the 1946 Protocol or `Paris Protocol'. Under this Protocol all functions assigned under the several conventions to organs of the new defunct League of Nations were transferred to the corresponding organs of the United Nations Organization. Thus all the functions of the old Opium Advisory Committee were assumed by the new Commission on Narcotic Drugs. The Commission has since concentrated on improvement of the existing treaty system and efficient national control wherever necessary.

33. New Potentials

From the information screened above, it is clearly evident that Cannabis is highly plastic, inasmuch it produces forms and varieties in accordance to operating influences of climate and soil. There are many factors which require detailed investigations (somatic or nuclear) regarding production of resins and anti-bacterial constituents in forms, growing in tropical and temperate regions.

Questions of sex fertility, its interdependence to photoperiodism and saltation, auxin development within the plant, is far from complete.

The plant appears to be an excellent tool for tracing biochemical pathways and chemical transformations, etc.

Furthermore, as Mikuriya[238] states "Medicine in the Western World has forgotten almost all it once knew about therapeutic properties of *Cannabis* (Marihuana).

Analgesia, anticonvulsant action, appetite stimulation, ataraxia, antibiotic properties and low toxicity were described throughout medical literature, beginning in 1839 when O' Shaughnessy introduced *Cannabis* into the Western pharmacopoeia.

As these findings were reported throughout Western Medicine, *Cannabis* attained wide use.

Cannabis therapy was described in most pharmacopoeial texts as a treatment for a variety of disease conditions.

During the second half of the 1800's and in the present century, medical researchers in some measure corroboratee the early reports of the therapeutic potentials of *Cannabis*. In addition, much laboratory research has been concerned with bioassay, determination of the mode of action, and attempts to solve the problems of insolubility in water and variability of strength among different Cannabis specimens.

'Recreational' smoking of *Cannabis* in the twentieth century and the resultant restrictive federal legislation in the United States have functionally ended all medical uses of Marihuana.

In the light of such assets as minimal toxicity, no build up of tolerance, no physical dependence, and minimal autonomic disturbance immediate major clinical re-investigation of *Cannabis* preparations....be made in the management of pain, chronic neurologic diseases, convulsive disorders, migraine, headache, anorexia, mental illness, and bacterial infections.

Summary

This review on the Genus Cannabis reflects information gathered from various disciplines, namely its taxonomy, complete morphology with newer additions of knowledge in recent years, on cultivation, ecology, production and utilization, Physiology, Flower-sex expression, sex differentiation, embryology, chromosomes, pollination endosperm, germination, seed oil, commercial fibres, anatomy, pests, entomology, virus and bacteria, fungi, diseases, insecticides, narcotics produced, chemical constituents, identification of Indian *Cannabis*, chemical tests, microscopic tests, biological evaluation, pharmacognosy, mode of consumption, addiction, newer chemical investigations, toxicity, reaction of drug on Man, pharmacology, psychiatry, allergy, antibiotic, antibacterial, international control and new potentials.

References

1. Abelson, P.H. Science, 159. (3820): 1187, (1968).
2. Adams, E.W. Practitioner, 129 : 234, 390, (1932).
3. Adams, R. and B.R. Baker. J. Am. Chem. Soc. 62 : 2401, (1940).
4. Adams, R. and B.R. Baker and R.R. Wearn. J. Am. Chem. Soc. 62: 2204 (1940).
5. Adams, R. D.C. Pease C.K. Cain and J.H. Clark. J. Am. Chem. Soc. 62: 2402, (1940).
6. Adams, R. C.K. Cain, W.D. Mc Phee and R.B. Wearn. J. Am. Chem. Soc. 63 : 2209, (1941).
7. Adams, R. Harvey Lectures. 37 : 168. (1942).
8. Adams, R. Bull. New York. Acad. Med. 18 : 705-29, (1942).
9. Adams, R.M. Harfenist and S. Loewe. J. Am. Chem. Soc. 71 : 1624, (1949).
10. Aguas da Silva, T. Maria, E.A. Carlini, Cuwe, K. Friedhelm : Psychoparmacologia 13(4) : 332-40, (1968).
11. Agurell, Stid-Nilsson, M. Inger, Finn Sandberg : Svensk. Farm. Tidskr. 72(20) : 662-70, (1968).
12. Ahluwalia, K.S. B.P.C. plants and their Indian substitutes. Govt. of India, Jamnagar, (1962).
13. Alexander, H.G. Narcotics in India and South Asia. Williams and Norgate Ltd. London. (1930).
14. Alexandrov, W.G. and Alexandrova, O.G.; Planta 7 : 340-346, (1929).
15. Allavena, D. Sementi elette, 7(3) : 26-35, (1961).
16. Allavena, D. Ital. agric. 99 : 237-53, (1962).
17. Allavena D. Sementi elette, 10 : 20-26, (1964).
18. Allport, N.L. The chemistry and pharmacy of vegetable drugs. George. Newness Ltd. London. p. 133-136, (1942).
19. Ammanus, J. Strip. Rar. Imp. Ruth, 174, (1939).
20. Anderson, G.S.D. Boston. Med. and Surg. J. 67 : 427-430 (1863).
21. Angelo, St. J. Allen, L.Y. Yatsu and Aaron. M. Attschul; Arch. Biochem. Biophys. 124 (1/3) : 199-205, (1968).
22. Angelo, St. J. Allen, Ann. Arbor. Mich. Order. 68-115 : 168, (1954).
23. Annoymous, Bull. Narcotics 2(2) : 32-54, (1950).
24. Annoymous, Bull. Narcotics 8(4) : 6-12, (1956).
25. Annoymous, Bull Narcotics 13(2) : 42-43, (1961).
26. Annoymous, Can. Med. Ass. J. 97(22) : 1359-1361, (1967).
27. Annoymous, Lancet. 1 : 139-140, (1969).
28. Antoniani, C. Ann. Accad. naz. Agric. Bologana. 73 : 255-282, (1963).
29. Aramaki, H. Tomiyasu, N. Yoshimura. Hidetoshi Tsukamoto. Hisao. Esei. Kagakru 14(5) : 262-5, (1968).
30. Arinstejn, A.I. and A.I. Pelipenko. Agrobiologija. 2 : 298-301, (1959).
31. Arnoux, M. Ann. Amel. Plantes. 13 : 27-49, (1963).
32. Ashe, A.L. Econ. Bot. 2(2) : 158-169, (1948).
33. Atal. C.K. Econ. Bot. 15 : 133-9, (1961).

34. Baden-Powel. Pb. Prod. 292-3, 504-7, (1968).
35. Baker, A.A. and E.G. Leucas. Lancet 1 : 148, (1969).
36. Bail, G.R. and L. Lazi. Brit. Jour. Pharm. and Pharmacol. 20(10) : 768-799, (1968).
37. Barloy, J. C.R. Acad. Agric. Fr. 48 : 194-201, (1962).
38. Barloy, J. and J. Pelhate, Ann. Epiphyt. 13 : 117-49, (1962).
39. Bary de, A. Comparative Anatomy of the vegetative organs of the Phanerogams and Ferns. Clarendon Press. Oxford, (1884).
40. Baudelaire, Ch. Less Paradis, artificiels, Poulet-Malassis, Paris, (1860).
41. Becker, H.S. Outsiders. Studies in the sociology of Deviance, Free Press. 41-58, (1953).
42. Bell, J. Boston. Med. and Surg. J. 56 : 209-16. 229-36, (1957).
43. Bellini, P. Ann. Sper. Agrar. 14 : 773-95, (1960).
44. Berkman, A.H. Seedling anatomy of *Cannabis sativa* L. Ph. D. Thesis Univ. Chicago, (1936).
45. Betts, T.J. and P.J. Holloway, J. Pharm. and Pharmacol. 19 : 975-1025, (1967).
46. Bergel, F. A.L. Morrison, H. Rinderknecht, A.R. Todd, A.D. Mac. Donald and G. Woofle. J. Chem. Soc. 286, (1943).
47. Birch, E.A. Lancet. 1 : 625, (1889).
48. Biswas, S.K. Gosh's Pharmacology Materia Medica and therapeutics. Hilton & Co. p. 1014, (1957).
49. Biswas, Birmingham University 32nd Annual Report on Research and Pub. (Sess. 1960-61). 144, (1961).
50. Bocsas, I. Kiserl. Kozlem. 52/A(3) : 135-42, (1959).
51. Boscsa, I. Novenytermeles. 10 : 43-50, (1961).
52. Bocsa, I. and G.L. Farkas. Phyton. Argentina. 16 : 189-93, (1961).
53. Bosca, I. Magy. tud. Akad. Agrartud. Oszt. Kozl. No. 1/3 : 65-84, (1958).
54. Bocsa, I and B. Simon, Novenytermeles. 13 : 21-26, (1964).
55. Bozner, M. Rostlinna. Vyroba. 6 : 121-30, (1960).
56. Bouhuys, A.A. Barbero, S.E. Lindell, S.A. Roach and R.S.F. Schiling. Arch. Environ. Health 14(4) : 533-544, (1967).
57. Bouquet, J. Bull. Nar. 2(4) : 14-30, (1950).
58. Bouquet, J. Bull. Nar. 3(1) : 22-45, (1951).
59. Bose, B.C. and B. Mikerji, Ind. J. Med. Res. 33 : 265, (1945).
60. Bredemann. G. Zeltschr. Pflanzensucht. 12 : 259-268, (1926).
61. Breslawetz, L. Ber. Deut. Bot. Gesell. 44 : 498-502, (1926).
62. Brodie, I. and B. Sen Gupta. Bull. Indian. Industr. Res. 10 : 19, (1943).
63. Bromberg, W. Am. J. Psychiat. 19 : 303-330, (1934).
64. Bromberg, W. J. Am. Med. A. 113 : 4-12, (1939).
65. Buchannan-Hamilton. Stat. Acc. Dinaj. 207, (1833).
66. Burger Alfred. Drugs effecting the central nervous system. Vol. 2. Marcel. Dekker. Inc. New York. p. 347, (1968).
67. Briosi, G. and F. Tognini. Att. Ist. Bot. Pavia. Ser. 11, 3 : 91-209, (1994).
68. Briosi, G. and F. Tognini. Atti. Ist. Bot. Pavia. Ser. II, 4 : 155-329, (1897).
69. Boyd, E.S. and D.A. Merritt. Arch. Internat. de Pharmacodynamie er de Therapie. 153 : 1-12, (1965).
70. Caddy, B. and F. Fish. J. Chromatog. 31 : 584-7, (1967).
71. Cahn, R.S. J. Che. Soc. 986, (1930).
72. Cahn, R.S. J. Chem. Soc. 630, (1931).
73. Cahn, R.S. J. Chem. Soc. 1342, (1932).

74. Cahn, R.S. J. Chem. Soc. 1400, (1933).
75. Candolle de, A. Origin of cultivated plants. D. Appleton and Co., (1885).
76. Cajlahjan, M.H. V.G. Kocankov, and V.P. Zamota, Fiziol. Rast. 7 : 340-3, (1960).
77. Carakushansky, G. R.L. Neu, and L.I. Gardner, Lancet. 1 : 150-151, (1969).
78. Cartwright, R.A. E.A.H. Roberts. Chem and Ind., 1389, 1954.
79. Chopra, R.N. and G.S. Chopra, Ind. J. Med. Res. Calcutta, Mem. 31 : 1. (1939).
80. Chopra, R.N. Ind. Med. Gar. 75 : 356, (1940).
81. Chopra, R.N. Science and Cultr. 5 : 761, (1940).
82. Chopra, R.N., Chopra, G.S. and I.C. Chopra. Ind. J. Med. Res. 30 : 155-71, (1942).
83. Chopra, R.N. B. Mukerji and I.C. Chopra. A treatise on tropical Therapeutics. U.N. Dhur and Sons Pvt. Ltd. Calcutta. (1954).
84. Chopra, I.C. and Chopra, R.N. Bull. Narcotics. 9(1) : 4-30, (1957).
85. Chopra, I.C.; K.L. Handa and L.D. Kapur. Indigenous Drugs of India. Calcutta, (1958).
86. Chopra, R.N.; S.L. Nayar, and I.C. Chopra. Glossary of Indian Medicinal Plants. CSIR. New Delhi, (1956).
87. Chopra, R.N. and I.C. Chopra. Drug addition. CSIR. (1965).
88. Chopra, R.N. S.L. Nayar and I.C. Chopra. Supplement to Glossary of Indian Medicinal Plants. CSIR, (1969).
89. C.C. Ital. Agric. 99 : 775-86, (1962).
90. C.E.C. Industrial fibres. Publ. Common. Econ. Cttee. 240. (1961).
91. C.E.C. Industrial fibres. Publ. Common. Econ. Cttee. 240. (1961).
92. C.E.C. CIBA, Foundation Study Group No. 21. ed. Hashish. Its chemistry and Pharmacology. Churchill. London. 45, 49, (1965).
93. Clark, L.D. and E.N. Nakashima. Am. J. Psychiat. 3 : 379-384, (1968).
94. Clark, Commission on Narcotic Druga. 11th Session UNESC. Doc. E/CN/7/ 286. Add. 12, (1960).
95. Clark, Commission on Narcotic Drugs. 16th Session Geneva, (1961).
96. Clark, Commander. Basic Hand Book. Drug abuse, game without winners, U.S.A., (1968).
97. Czechoslava. Faculty. Medicine. University Palacky. Olomouc. Acta. Univ. Palackianae. Olomucensis. Fac. Med. 43 : 111-124, (1966), (1967).
98. Conrad, K. and K. Mothes. Naturwissenchaften. 48 : 26-27, (1961).
99. Conrad, K. Flora Jena. 152 : 68.73, (1962).
100. Cordeiro de Farias, R. Bull. Narcotics. 7(2) : 5-19, (1955).
101. Crombie, L., R. Ponsford. Chem. Commun. 15 : 894-5, (1968).
101. Crooks, D.M., Bod Gaz. 95 : 209-239, (1933).
103. Cross, C.F. and E.J. Bevann. Researches on Cellulose II. Longmans. Green and Co. London, (1913).
104. Cunningham, D.D. Report of Indian Hemp Drugs Commission. 1893-4. Govt. Printing Office, Simla, India. 3 : 192-96, (1894).
105. Davidjan, G.G. Agro Biologija. 6 : 922-5, (1963).
106. davidjan, G.G. Tr. Priklad. Bot. Genet. Seleke, 35(2) : 222-8, (1963).
107. Davis, J.P. and H.H. Ramsey. Federat. Proc. 8 : 284, 85, 1949.
108. Davis, T.V.M., C.G. Farmilo and M. Osadchuk. Analyst. Chem. 35 : 751-5, (1963).
109. Davis, G.L. Systematic Embryology of the Angiosperms John Wiley and Sons., Inc. New York, (1966).
110. De Ropp. R.S. J. Amer. Pharm. ass. Sci. 49 : 756-8, (1960).

111. Dewey, L.H. 'Hemp' U.S. Dept. Agr. Yearbook. 283-346, (1913).
122. Dewey, L.H. The hemp. industry in the United States. U.S. Dept. Agr. Yearbook. 541-554, (1901).
113. Dioscorides. P. The Greek Herbal of Dioscorides. Ed. R.T. Gunther. Hafner. Pub. Co; New York. 390-91, (1959).
114. Dixon, W.E. Brit. Med. J. 2 : 1354, (1999).
115. *Action* : Doge, C.R. U.S. Dept. Agr. Fiber. Invest. Rep. 9 : 361, (1897).
116. Dodge, Recent developments in the treatment of paroled offenders addicted to narcotic drugs. U.S.A. Alabany, (1964).
117. Dutt. C. Mat. Med. Hindu. 235-41, (1900).
118. Dutt. C. In Psychopharmacological Agents Vol. I. (M. Gorden. Ed.) Academic, New York. 555-618, (1964).
119. Eddy, N.B. H. Halbach, Isbell. H. and M.H. Seevers. Psychoparmacology Bull. 3 : 1-12, (1966).
120. Eddy, N.B. Effects of alcohol and Cannabis during labor. JAMA. 94 : 1165, (1930).
121. Elfving, F. Jen. Zeit. f. Nat. 13 : 1-28, (1880) Quart. J. Micros. Sci. 20 : 1935, (1879).
122. Elfving, Evaluation of Dependence-producing Drugs. WHO. Tech. Rep. Ser. 287, (1964).
123. *Ewens, G.F.W.E.* Indian. Med. Gaz. 39 : 401-13, (1904).
124. Fahmy, I.R. and El. Keiy. C.R. XII. Cong. Internat. Pharm. 185, (1935).
126. Arnasworth, N.R. Science 162 : 1086-92, (1968).
127. Farnsworth, N.R. J. Amer. Pharm. Ass. 9(8) : 410-17, (1969).
128. Farnsworth, Res. Rept. Agri. Inst. Plant. Sciences and Crop. Husb. Div. Dublin. 75, (1961).
129. Ferri, F. Progr. agric. Bologna. 7 : 349-56, (1961).
130. Ferri, F. Progr. agric. Bologna, 7 : 764-5, (1961).
131. Ferri, F. Progr. agric. Bologna. 9 : 346-51, (1963).
132. Ferri, F. and C. Noviello. Phytopath. medit. 2 : 72-5, (1963).
133. Ferenczy, L. Gracza L. and I. Jakobey. Naturwissenchaften 45 : 188, (1958).
134. Flahault. C. Ann. Sci. Nat. Bot. Ser. VI. 6 : 1-168, (1978).
135. Fujita, M.H. Shimomura., E. Kuriyama, M. Schigehiro, and M. Akasu. Syoyakugaku. Zasshi. 21(1) : 57-64 (1967).
136. Fujita, F.A.O. World Fibre Survey. 131, (1947).
137. Gaoni. Y. and R. Mehoulam. Proc. Chem. Soc. 82 : 1646-7, (1964).
139. Ganatra, J.P. M.A. Patel, S. Satakopan and M.R. Shastri. Indian. Jr. Pharm. 30 (12) : 282, (1969).
140. Garriott, J.C., L.J. King, R.B. Forney and F.W. Hughes. Life Sci. 6(19. Pt. I.) : 2119-2128, (1967).
141. Garriott, J.C., R.B. Forney, F.W. Hughes, and A.B. Richards. Arch. Inst. Pharmacodyn. Ther. A.B. Richards. Arch. Inst. Pharmacodyn. Ther. 171 (2) : 425-434, (1968).
142. Gayer, H. ARch. Exptl. Pathol. Pharmakol. 129 : 312, (1928).
143. Geber. W.F. and L.C. Schramm. Toxicol. Appl Pharmacol. 14 : 276-282, (1969).
144. Ghosh, R., A.R. Todd and S. Wilkinson. J. Chem. Soc. 1121 : 1393, (1940).
145. Goidanich. Athos. Bol. Isab. Ent. Inst. Sup. Agrario. Bolgna. 1 : 37-64, (191928).
146. Goidanich, G. and F. Ferri. Phytopath. Z. 37 : 21-32, (1959).
147. Goddman, L.S. and A. Gilman. The pharmacological basis of Therapeutics. 2nd ed. Mac Millian. New York. 171, (1955).

148. Graff. H. Am. J. Psychiat. 125 : 152-153, (1969).
149. Grlic. Lj. Farm. Glasnik. 24 : 455-458, (1968).
150. Grossman. W. Ann. Internal. Med. 70 : 529-533, (1969).
151. Grossman, The control and treatment of narcotic use. U.S. Dept. of Health, Education and welfare, (1966).
152. Hamliton, H.C. Lescohier. A.W., and R.A. Perkins. J. Amer. Pharm. Assoc. 2 : 22-30, (1913).
153. Hanichirou, Aramaki, Naoko Tomiyasu, Hidetoshi Yoshimura, and Hisao Tasukamoto. Chem. Pharm. Bull. 16(5) : 822-826, (1968).
154. Hanin, M.D. Agro-biologija. 1 : 58-63, (1959).
155. Hayward, H.E. The structure of Economic plants Mac Millan Co. New York, (1938).
156. Hare, Hobart. Amory, Therap. Gaz. 11 : 225-28, (1887).
157. Hare, H.A. and W. Chrystie. A System of Practical Therapeutics. Philadelphia, (1892).
158. Heaysman, L.T., Walker, E. and D.T. Lewis, Analyst, 92 : 405-5, (1967).
159. Herich, R. and Priehradny, S. Bilogia. Bratishlava. 10 : 346-9, (1955), 11 : 111-15, (1956).
160. Herich, R. Biologia. Bratishlava. 11 : 220-4, (1956).
161. Herich, R. Acta. Fac. Rer. Nat. Univ. Comm. Bot. I : 419-25, (1956).
162. Herich, R. Phyton (Austria). 9 : 126-34, (1960).
163. Herich, R. Pol' nohospodarstvo. 8 : 193-9, (1961).
164. Herich, R. Nature. 188 : 599-600, (1960).
165. Herich, R. Physiol. Plant. 14 : 111-14, (1961).
166. Hesslor, F. Der Ayurveda des Susruta. F. Enke Erlangae. 1, 2, (1844, 1850).
167. Helop-Harrison, Y., and I, Woods. J. Linn. Soc. (Bot.) 56 : 290-3, (1959).
168. Heslop-Harrison, Y. Science, 132. 1943-4 (1960).
169. Heuser. O. Die. Hanfplanzen. Ed. J. Springer. Berlin, (1927).
170. Hiroko Shimomura, Michiko Shigehiro, Etsuko Kuriyama, and Mititi Fujita. Yakugaku Zasshi 87(1) : 1334-1341, (1967).
171. Hoernle, A.F. J. Asiatic Soc. Calcutta. 70 (I), (1901).
172. Hoernle, A.G. Central Asiatic manuscripts. J. asiatic Soc. of Bengal. 66 : 247, (1897).
173. Hoernle, A.G. Studies in the Medicine of Ancient India I. London., (1907).
174. Hopskins, J.F. A history of the Hemp. Industry in Kentucky Univ. of Kentucky Press. 240, (1951).
175. I.P.C. Indian Pharmaceutical Codex. Delhi, (1952).
176. I.P.C. Indigenous Drug Inquiry (Ed. R.N. Chopra). Central Indigenous Drugs Committee. Delhi, (1950).
177. I.P.L. Indian Pharmacopoeial List, (1946).
178. Jacob, A. and A.R. Todd. J. Nature. 145 : 350, (1940).
179. Jacob, A. and A.R. Todd. J. Chem. Soc. 649, (1940).
180. Janczewski, E. Ann. Sci. Nat. Bot. Ser. V. 20 : 162-201, *1874).
181. Janisevskij, F.V. Fiziol. Rast. 8 : 658-62, (1961).
182. Jain, S.K. Medicinal plants. National Book trust New Delhi, (1968).
183. Jeung. Haeng. Ree. Edon. Bot. 20 : 176-86, (1966).
184. Jimenez-Diaz, C., E. Lopez-Garcia ff. Lahoz, J. Ramirez-Guedes an d J.M. Ales. Rev. Clin. Espan. 103(3) : 182-188, (1966).
185. Kales, A., Heuser. G., Kales, J.D., W.H. Rickles, R.T. Rubin, M.B. Scharf, J.T. Ungerleider and W.D. Winter. Ann. Internal. Med. 70 : 591-614, (1969).

186. Kalinkevic, A.F. and G.V. Udovenko. Doklady. Akad. Nauk. S.S.S.R. 136 : 684-7, (1959).
187. Kalisevic, S.V. and N.V. Porohnevic. Fiziol. Rast. II. 206-9, (1964).
188. Kane, V., V. Razdan, K. Raj. J. Amer. Chem. Soc. 90 (23) : 6551-3, (1968).
189. Kechatov. E.A. Bull. Narcotics. 11(4) : 5, (1959).
190. Keeler. M. Amer. J. Psychiat. 124(5) : 674-677, (1967).
191. Kirtikar, K.R. Basu B.D. Indian Medicinal Plants. Vol. 4. Allahabad, (1934).
192. Kingston, K.R. Basu B.D. Indian Medicinal Plants. Vol. 4. Allahabad, (1934).
192. Kingston, C.R. and P.L. Kirk. Analyst. Chem. 33 : 1794-5, (1961).
193. Kohler. D. Planta. 56 : 150-73, (1961).
194. Korte, F. and H. Sieper. Liebigs. Ann. Chem. 630 : 71, (1960).
195. Korte, F. and H. Sieper. J. Chromatog. 14 : 178-83, (1964).
196. Korte, F. and H. Sieper. in Hashish : Its Chemistry and Pharmacology. (Ciba Foundation Study Group. 21 ed.). Churchill. London. 15, (1965).
197. Krejci, Z., M. Horak, and F. Santavy. Pharmazie. 14 : 349, (1959).
198. Kundu, B.C. J. Indian. Bot. Soc. 21 : 93-128, (1942).
199. Kundu, B.C. and R.D. Preston. Proc. Roy. Soc. B. 128 : 214-31, (1940).
200. Lacznska-Hulewiczowa, T. Acta. Soc. bot. Polon. 26 : 515-49, (1957).
201. Langlet. O.F. Svensk. Bot. Tidskr. 21 : 397-422, (1927).
202. Laskowska, R. Nature. 192 : 147-8, (1961).
203. Lelaksi, P. Delt. agrotik. Trap. 117 : 19, (1960).
204. Lewin, L. Phantastika. George Stilke. Berling. (1924).
206. Lewin, L. Phantastica. Narcotic and stimulating drugs, their use and abuse. Routledge and Paul Kegan. London. (1964).
207. Limberk, J. Biol. Plant. Prague. 1 : 176-86, (1959).
20.8. Litardiere de, R. La Cellule. 35 : 21-25, (1925).
209. Litardiere Lilly's Hand Book of Pharmacy and Therapeutics, Eli. Lilly and Col. Indanapolis. 32, (1898).
210. Loewe, S. J. Pharmacol. Exptl. Therap. 88 : 154-61, (1946).
211. Lowew, S. Arch. Exptl. Pathol. Pharmakol. 211 : 175, (1950).
212. Lopez-Merino, v., A. Romar. Mico, R. Liopis-Llombart, R. Flores-Marco and A. Barbero-Carnicero. Med. Segur. Trab. (Madrid.) 14 (56) : 51-61, (1966).
213. Lubbock, J. Seedlings. 2.D. Appleton and Co. (1892).
214. Ljusinskij, V.V. Zasc. Rast. vred. Bolez. 7(10) : 24-25, (1959).
215. Manninger, I. Bocsa, I. and Z. Klement. Novenytermeles. 8 : 259-72, (1959).
216. Manolache. C., I . Sandru and Em. Romascu. Probl. Agr. 6 : 68-72, (1966).
217. Marks, V. and P.A.L. Chapple. Brit. J. Addict. 62 (Ū : 189-195, (1967).
218. Marshall, C.R. JAMA; 31 : 882-91, (1898).
219. Martinec, T. and M. Felklova. Pharmazie. 14 : 276-9, (1959).
220. Martinec, T. and M. Felklova. Pharmazie. 14 : 279-81, (1959).
221. Martin, L.D. M. Smith, C.G. Farmilo. Nature. 191 : 774-6, (1961).
223. Mattison, J.B. ST. Louis Med. and Surg. J. 61 : 265-71, (1891).
224. Matthews, J.M. The textile Fibres. John. Wiley and Sons, (1911).
225. Matthews, Mayor's Committee on Marihuana. The Marihuana problem in the City of New York, Jaques. Cattell. Lancaster. Pa., (1944).
226. McMeens. R.R. Report of the Committee on *Cannabis indica*. Transactions of the 15th Annual Meeting of the Ohio State Medical Society, Follett. Foster and Co. Columbus, Ohio. 75-100, (1860).
227. Mcphee, H.C. Jour. Agr. Res. 28 : 1067-1080, (1924).
228. Mcphee, H.C. Jour. Agr. Res. 31 : 935-943, (1925).

229. McGlothlin, W.H. New Physicia. 18 : 196-202, (1969).
230. Mechoulam, R. and Y. Shvo. Tetrahedron. 19 : 2073, (1943).
231. Mechoulam. R. Israel. J. Chem. I : 57-8, (1963).
232. Mechoulam. R. Benzvi. Z.Y. Gaoni. Tetrahedron. 24(16) : 5615-24, (1968).
234. Menzel. M.Y. Bull. Torrey. Bot. Club.
235. Miras, C.J. in Hasish. Its chemistry and Pharmacology. (Ciba. Foundation Study Group No. 21). Churchill. London, (1965).
237. Mikuriya, T.H. Econ. Bot. 21 : 230-4, (1967).
238. Mikuriya, T.H. Calif. Med. 110 : 34-40, (1969).
239. Mitchell. J. Bull. Narcotics. 8(3) : 9-14, (1961).
240. Mitiiti Fujita, Hiroko Shimomura, Etsuko Kuriyama, Michiko Shigehiro and Michinori Akasu. Syokakugaku Zasshi. 21(1) : 57-64, (1967).
241. Moon. John. B. Sir William Brooke. O'Shaughnessy-the foundation of fluid therapy and the Indian telegraph service. New Eng. J. of Med. 276 : 283-84, (1867).
242. Murphy, H.B.M. Bull. Narcotics. U.N. Dept. Social Affaris, 15 : 15, (1963).
243. Mukerji, B. Indian Pharmaceutical Code. CSIR. New Delhi, (1953).
244. Myers. S.A. and D.F. Caldwel. New Physician. 18 : 212-215, (1969).
245. Nadkarni, K.M. Indian Materia Medica, Bombay, (1954).
246. Nevinnyh. V.A. Agrobiologija. 2kg 205-12, (1962).
247. Nigam, M.C. Cand. J. Chem. 43 : 3372-6, (1965).
248. Noirfalise. A.J. Pharm. Belg. 23(7-8) : 387-99, (1968).
249. Novak, I., Buzas, G. and L. Toth. Pharmazie. 17 : 166-73, (1962).
250. Novak, I. Buzas, G. and L. Toth. Pharmazie. 17 : 95-8, (1962).
251. Novak. I., Haznagy, a. and K. Szendrei. Pharmazie. 17 : 294-7, (1962).
252. O'Shaughnessy, W.B. Trans. Med. and Phy. Soc. Bengal. 71-102, (1838-40); 421-61 (1842).
253. Olser. W. and T. McCrae, Principles and practice of Medicine, 8th Ed. D. Appleton and Co., New York. 1089., (1916).
254. Pamplona, M. Ramos. A.C. An. Fac. Farm. Univ. Recife. 8/9 : 65-76, (1965)., (1966).
255. Parker, C.S. and F. Wrigley. J. and Mental Science. 96 : 176-79, (1950).
256. Paskovic, F. Tekstil. 7(2) : 105-24, (1958).
257. Paskovic, Parliament Paper. Ganja and other drugs in India. March 3, (1893).
258. Phatak, H.C. and S.K. Batra. Indian. J. Microbiol. 6(3/4) : 49-50, (1966).
259. Pond, D.A. J. Neurol. Neurosurg. Psychiat. 11 : 271-79, (1948).
260. Prain, I. Rept. Cult. and Uses of Ganja. Goct. of India. Calcutta, (1898).
261. Pursoglove, J.W. Tropical Crops-Dictoyledons I. Longmans. 40-44, (1968).
262. Rabinovic, A.S., Ajzeman, B.E. and S.I. Zelepuha. J. Microbiol. Kiev. 21(2) : 40-8, (1959).
263. Radosevic, A., Kupinic, M. and Grlic Lj. Nature, 195 ; 1007-9, (1962).
264. Ram, M. Ann. bot. Lond. 24 : 79-82, (1960).
265. Ranquini, J.H. Bull. inst. Catalana his. nat. (2) 8 : 71-76, (1928).
266. Ratnam, E.V. J. Ceylon. Brit. Med. Assoc. 13 : 30-34, (1916).
267. Ratnam, Report. Hemp. Drugs Commission. Govt. of India (1893-94).
268. Rantam, Report. traffic in Opium and other dangerous drugs. Govt. of India, (1944).
269. Ratnam, Report of the Committee on legislative activities. JAMA. 108 : 2214-15, (1937).
270. Redersen, A. Bot. Tidsskr. 62(2/3) : 85-122, (1966).

271. Renolds, J.R. Lancet. i kg 637-38, (1890).
272. Robinson, V. An essay in Hasheesh, Historical and Experimental. L.H. Ringer, New York, (1912).
273. Roll, E.J. and C.D. Stafford. Guy's Hospital Rept.
274. Rousinov. K-S. and Athana-Sova-Shopova. C.R. Acad. Bulg. Sci. 19(4) : 333-336, (1966).
275. Sampaio. C.A.M. A.I. Lapa and J.R. Valle. J. Pharm. Pharmacol. 19(8) : 552-554, (1967).
276. Santavy, F. acta. Univ. Palackianae. Olomuc. Fac. Med. 35 : 5, (1964).
277. Sasman, Marty. J.N.J. Med. Soc. 35 : 51-52, (1938).
278. Savelli, R. Ach. Botan. 4 : 128-137, (1928).
279. Savelli, R. Arch. Bot. Sist. Fitogeogr. e. Ganet. 4(2) : 128-137, (1928).
280. Schilling, E. Ber. Dtsch. bot. Ges. 41 : 121-7, (1923).
281. Schaffner, J.H. Ecology, 7 : 315-325, (1926).
282. Schaffner, J.H. Am Jour. Bot. 15 : 77-85, (1928).
283. Schaffner, J.H. Amer. Nat. 64(693) : 367-379, (1930).
284. Schultz. O.E. and G. Haffner, Arch., Pharm. 291 : 391, (1958).
285. Schultz, O.E. Z. Naturforsch. 141 : 98, (1959).
286. Schultz, O.E. Plant Medica. 12 : 37, (1964).
287. Schultes, R.E. Science. 163 : 245-54, (1969).
288. Sircar, R. Misc. Bull. I.C.A.R. 66 : 33, (1948).
289. Spaldon, E. Laskos, J. and J. Vasuta. Sborn. vys. sk. Pol'no hosp. v. Nitre-agron. Fak. 3 : 39-53, (1961).
290. Spulak, von. F., Claussen, U., Fehlhaber, H.W., F. Korte. Tetrahedron. 24 : 15, (1968).
291. Stant, M.Y. Ann. Bot. Lond. 27 : 185-96, . 63).
292. Shoyama, Yukihiro, Fujita, T., T. Yamauchi, I. Nishioka. Chem. Pharm. Bull (Tokyo). 16(6) 1157-8, (1968).
293. Stankovic, L. Letopisnauc. Rad. Novi. Sad. 3 : 156-61, (1959).
294. Steinmetz, E.F. Materia Medica Vegetabilis. Part I 101, (1954).
295. Stevens, A.A. Modern Materia Medica and Therapeutics. W.B. Saunders and Co. Philadelphia. 77-78, (1903).
296. Stockings, G.T. Brit. Med. J. 1 : 918-22, (1947).
297. Strasburger; E. Histolog. Beitr. 7 ; 1-124, (1909).
298. Sudi, J. Bot. Gaz. 123 : 265-72, (1962).
299. Stuart, K.L.W. Indian. Med. J. 12(3) : 156-160, (1963).
300. Sushruta Samhita. Sushrutacharya. Nirnaya Sagar Press Bombay, (1939).
301. Suckling, C.W. Brit. Med. J. 2 : 12, (1881).
302. Szilagyi, L. Novenytermeles. 12 : 143-6, (1963).
303. Szilagyi, Sharangadhara Samhita. Sharangadharacharya Nirnaya Sagar Press, Bombay, (1932).
304. Taylor, E.C. K. Lenard and Y. Shavo. J. Am. Chem. Soc. 88 : 367-9, (1966).
305. Terry, C.E. and M. Pellens. The Opium problem. Bureau of Social Hygiene. Inc. New York. 53-93, (1928).
306. Thompson, L. J. and R.C. Proctor. N. Carolina. Med. J. 14 : 520-23, (1953).
307. Tieghem, van. P. and H. Douliot. Ann. Sci. Nat. Bot. Ser. VII. 8 : 1-656, (1888).
308. *Tippo, H. Bot*. Gaz. 100 : 1-99, (1938).
309. Tkalic, pp. Zasc, Rast. Vred. Bolez. 6(8) : 24-5, (1961).
310. Tkalic, U.S. Treasury Dept. Bureau of Narcotics, Traffic in Opium and other dangerous drugs for the year ended Dec. 31, (1965). U.S. Printing Office, Washington, 55-56, (1966).

311. Todd. A.R. Endeavour. 48, (1953).
312. Tournois, J. C.R. Acad. Sci. Paris. 153 : 1160-1162, (1911.
313. Tournois, J. Ann. Sci. nat. Bot. (9) : 19, (1914).
314. Treggi, G. Ann. Sper. agrar. 14 : 1003-7, (1960).
315. Treggi, G. Plant and Soil. 15 : 291-4, (1961).
316. Tudosie, A.D. and V. Topar. Grad. Via. Liv. 10(3) : 20-22, (1961).
317. Unwin, J.R. Can Med. Assoc. J. 98 : 449-453, (1968).
318. Valle, J.R. Lapa, A.J., Barros and G. Glauce. J. Pharm. Pharmacol. 20(10) : 798-9, (1968).
319. Vieira, F. J. Amaral, M.B. Agular, J.W. Alencar, A. Prado-Seabra, B.M. Tursch, and J. Leclercq. Psychopharamacologia. 10(4) : 361-362, (1967).
320. Vincent, M. and P.A.L. Chapple. Brit. J. addict. 62 (Ū) : 189-195, (1967).
321. Watt. J.M. Bull. Narcotics. 13 (3) : 9-14, (1961).
322. Watt. G. The Commercial product of India. London. 249, 163, (1908).
323. Watt. P. and M.G. Breyer-Brandwijk. The medicinal and poisonous plants of Southern and Eastern africa. 2nd Ed. Livingstone. Edinburgh. 759, (1962).
324. Watt. P. Estimated World Requirements of Narcotic Drugs in 1964 (U.N. New York), (1964).
325. Walton, R.P. Marihuana, America's New drug problem. 1018, 86-157. J.B. Lippincott. New York, (1938).
326. Waring, E.J. Practical Therapeutics. Lindsay and Blakiston, Philadelphia. 157-61, (1874).
327. Weitz, R. and C. Dardanne. Bull. Sci. Pharmacol. 31 : 321, (1924).
328. Wettstein, R. von. Flora. 118-119. 600-604, (1925).
329. Wettstein, R. von. Hand buch. der systematischen Botanik. Leipzig. Wien., (1924).
330. Winge, O. The pollination and fertilization process in *Humulus lupulus* and *H. Japanicus*. C.R. trav. Lah. Carlsberg. 11, (1914).
331. Winton, A.L. and Winton, K.B. The structure of composition of foods., (1935).
332. Wollner, H.J., J.R. Machett, J. Levine and S. Loewe. J. Am. Chem. Soc. 64 : 26, (1942).
333. Wood, H.C. Jr. Proc. Am. Philos. Soc. 11 : 226, 232, (1869)-(1870).
334. Wood, G.B. and F. Bache. The Dispensatory of the United States of America. 12th Ed. J.B. Lippincott, Philadelphia. 379-82, (1866).
335. Wood, G.B. White House Conference on Narcotic and Drug Abuse. Washington Govt. Printing Office, (1963).
336. Wood, G.B. *Cannabis*. Wealth of India. Raw materials II : 58-64, (1950).
337. Ymauchi, Tatsuo, Shoyama Yukihiro, Matsuo Yoko, Nishioka Itsuo, Chem. Pharm. Bull. (Tokyo). 16(6) : 1164-5, (1968).
338. Yawger, N.S. Am. J. Med. Sci. 195 : 351-357, (1938).
339. Yegna, N., Iyer, A.K. Field Crops of India. Madras. 479, (1944).
340. Youngken, H.W. The Text book of Pharmacognosy. Blakistan Co. Philadelphia. 273, (1947).
341. Yukihiro, S., F. Toshio. Y. Tatsuo, N. Itsuo. Chem. Pharm. Bull. (tokyo). 16(6) : 1157-8, (1968).
342. Yukaka Jono. Acta. Scholae. Med. Univ. Imp. Kioto. 13(3) : 211-238, (1931).
243. Zander, A. Flora Jena. 123 : 191-218, (1928).
344. Zemljanuhin, A.A. and Sensina, S.V. Fiziol. Rast. 8 : 213-19, (1961).
345. Zinger, N. Flora 85 : 189-292, (1898).
346. Zinberg. N.E. and A.T. Weil. Nature. 226 : 119-123, (1970).

V

DATURA

This is the third plant, commonly referred to in Hindu Medical texts and religious books.

Datura has been used as a narcotic, since time immemorial. Plant is termed as "Shiva-shekhara", because the flowers and fruits, are blessed by lord Siva, for attaining mental peace.

The term *"Datura"* is derived from the Sanskrit word *"Dhatura"*, which refers to the capsules of *D. metal.*[1]

The hypnotic effects following the ingestion of almost any part of the *Datura* species has long been dreaded with fear. There effects have been utilized both in the Old world, Asia and in America in religious ceremonies; in oracular divination or in the forecasting of future events. All species of the genus *Datura* seem to possess the same properties to quite a large extent.

Indians have long been familiar with the narcotic and intoxicating properties of this drug-plant, (*D. metel*), so much so, some unscrupulous individuals (thieves and thugs) use to stupefy their victims by introduction the seeds of the *Datura* in their food.

In South America, some wild tribes make use of these plants to induce partial intoxication to their un-wanted women-folks and slaves, to deaden there senses before burying them alive, with their dead husbands or masters. Extracts from bark leaves and seeds of these plants have been used in shamanistic rites and practices. The Aztec Indians[2] use *Datura meteloides*, which they call as 'the mague plant' or "Gloliuheui". The entire plant leaves roots flowers seeds are used by Aztecs against all diseases, either applied as an ointments to wounds and cuts; in cases of paralysis, and for its narcotic effects. Drinks prepared from these plants were also used in various ceremonies by priests or medicine men, to enable them to communicate with the spirits. The drug provokes various effects, depending probably on the dose taken.

In commonly causes phantasmic visions or induce oracular prophecies. The Aztecs, consider the seeds of this plant sacred, make sacrificial offerings to them, and keep them on their altars.

Plant : (*D. metel*) The plant[3] is a woody herb growing to a height of 1.5 m, with many divaricate succulent spreading branches. Each shoot in the flowering region has two leaves, terminated by a flower. The two leaves have exillary buds which later develop into opposite pair of branches (dichasium). These subtending leaves, how-ever are not found in their correct position. They become free from their axillary branches at the place where first ones are produced, so in a mature shoot the flowers are borne singly.

Root : Main root (tap-root) as deep as 30 cm with many secondary and tertiary branches.

Stem Erect herbaceous, when young and slightly woody at maturity. In old plants surfaces are green with dark violet shades, glabrous, slightly puberulose, in young parts branching divaricate.

Leaf: Simple, ramal 9-20 cm long and 5-16 cm broad ovate apex acute, margin entire when young, irregularly lobed at maturity, inequilateral at base, main and side nerves conspicuous, 4 to 5 on each side of central vein. Petiole 8-20 cm long puberulose, slightly channeled at the base.

Venation unicostate, reticulate and are stipulate, glaucous, green above and palegreen below.

Inflorescense : Dichasial cyme, flower solitary, ebracteate, pedicellate, complete, actinomorphic, hermaphrodite and hypogynous. Colour: Yellowish, or dull white with violet tinge, pedicel 1.0-1.5 cm long, stout with 2 small protuberances at the base, flowers slightly inclined and infundibuliform. Calyx: 5 lobed, gamosepalous, tubular, turgid about 5.0 to 6.5 cm in length, teeth 5, triangular 1.3-29 cm long, triangular acute, sepaloid; aestivation valvate and hypogynous. *Corolla* : 1-lobed. gamopetalous 15-17 cm long and 8-9 cm across the mouth, dull white, pinkish in the folds, violet at ridges and on the lobes, limbs 5-6 short, acute with dilated lobes and a short tail in the middle of each intervening sinus, tips slightly hooked. *Androecum*: stamens 5, epipetalous, free part 4-5-6.5 cm filaments slender glabrous, fused part pubescent, much raised sharply channeled, another 1.2 to 1.3 cm long, obtuse basifixed; dehiscence longitudinal, by a slit; pollen (average size) 0.646 u in diameter. *Gynsecium* : Bicarpellary, syncarpous, superior, ovary with axile placentation, placenta swollen, ovules many, ovary purplish, clothed with numerous blunt tubercles, bilocular but becomes tetra-locular, due to the ingrowth of the placenta, ovary slightly obliquely placed, style 11.5 to 13.0 cm long, stigma bilobed. *Fruit* : A capsule, nodding, on curved pedicel, sub-globose 3-4 cm across, supported on a reflexed calyx base, covered with numerous short conical tubercles, around each tubercle an area is marked along with capsule usually splits open. Dehiscence setifragal. Seeds numerous, olive brown, closely packed, compressed reniform, smooth, size 4-5 mm long, and 3.9-3.2 mm broad, white caruncle, place towards the concave side of the seed, embryo curved. Pollination, entomophilous.

Chemistry and Pharmacology

Atropine, hyoscyamine and hyoscine, alkaloids from *Datura* have their use in modern medicine.

Atropine is used for causing dilation of the pupil of eye. All the species of *Datura* contain alkaloids of the tropane class. Furthermore, apart from cusco-hygrine, all the alkaloids of *Datura* are derivatives of tropane (i)

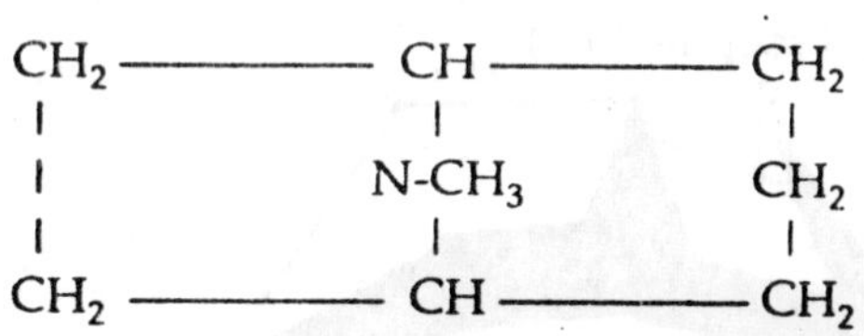

(I)

The most abundant alkaloid is hyoschyamine (II)

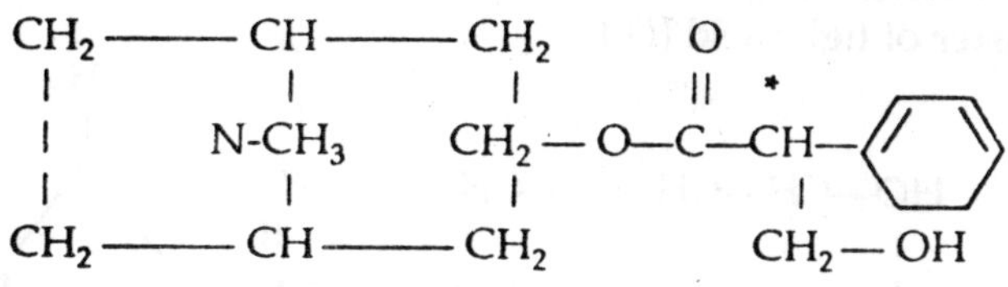

(II)

(This alkaloid has an asymmetric carbon denoted by an astrik).

The optically active form is known as hyoscyamine and the racemic mixture is atropine. Like most of the tropane lakaloids, hyoscyamine is an ester readily breaking at the O-CO- bound, producing an alcohol tropine, and an acid, tropic acid.

Formula III represents the established sterechemical relation of the atoms in tropine.

Nor-hyoscyamine (VI) is a minor alkaloid differing from hyoscyamine by absence of the methyl group attached to nitrogen.

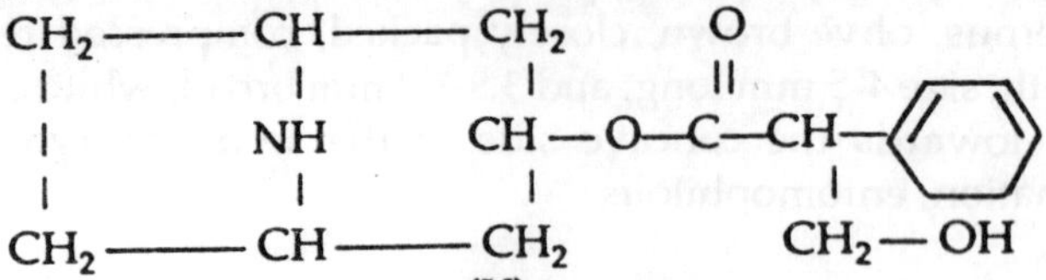

(V)

Hyoscine (VI) is also known as scopolamine

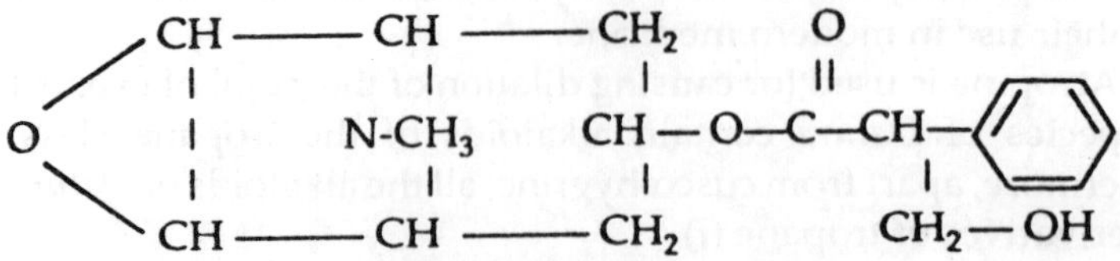

is wide-spread alkaloid in this genus. It is an ester of tropic acid and the alcohol socpine (VII).

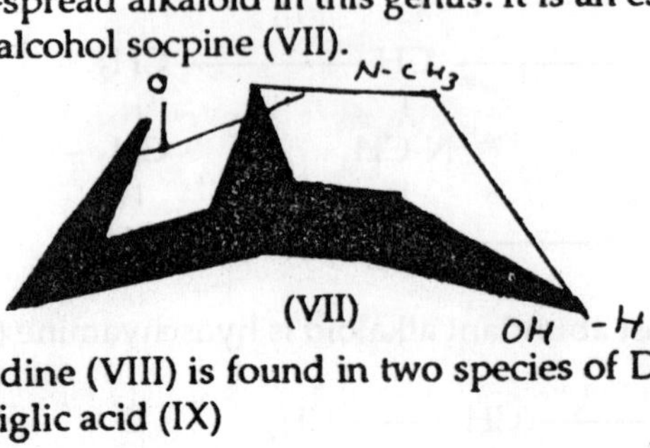

(VII)

Meteloidine (VIII) is found in two species of Datura and is an easter of tiglic acid (IX)

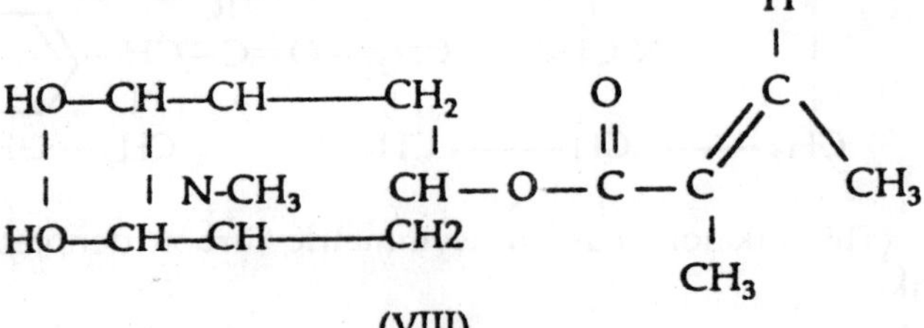

(VIII)

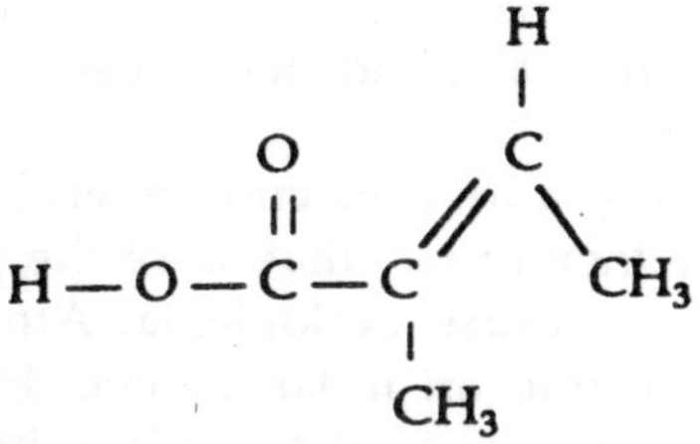

(IX)

and teloidine (X)

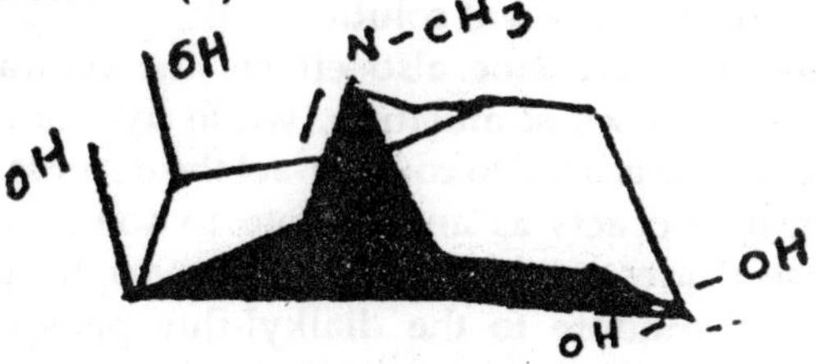

(X)

From roots on alkaloid is also isolated. It present structure (XI) given below and is 3,6-ditighylteloidine.

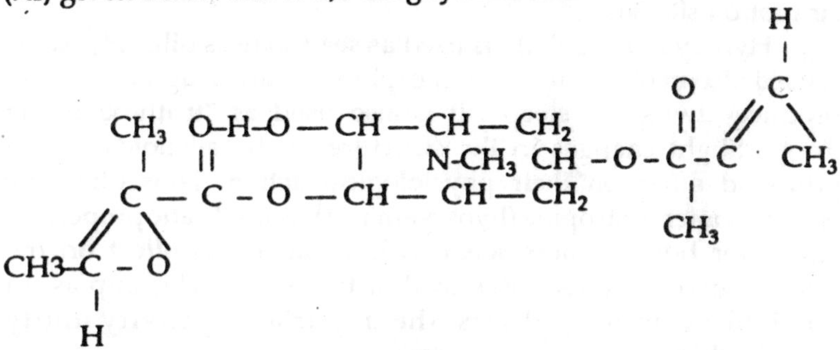

(XI)

Cuseo-hygrine (XII) has also been detected in the roots of several *Datura* species.

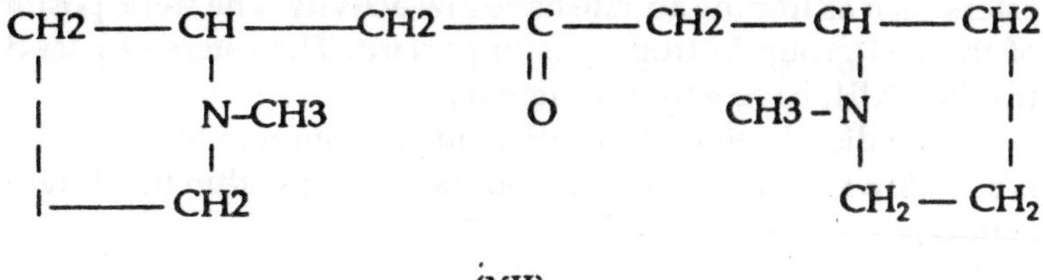

(XII)

Tropane ring is absent, but it may be related to other alkaloids biogenetically. Chemistry of these alkaloids have been discussed by Henry[4], Holmes,[5] Foder[6] etc.

A tropine, hyoscyamine and hyoscine referred to as mydriatic alkaloids, because they cause dilation of the pupil of the eye (mydriasis). They also cause cycloplegia. Atropine is used in opthalmology, for resting an inflamed eye. Hyoscine produces, the same effect on the eye as atropine, but its effects are weaker and of shorter duration. It is frequently used as hydrochloride in 1 to 2 percent solutions.

A tropine and hyoscine also effects the central nervous system. Atropine causes stimulation, while hyoscine acts as a depressant. Atropine is used to counter-act the depression caused by morphine. It also acts as an antidote to some highly toxic phosphate insecticides, such as tetra-ethyl-pyrophosphate. It is also used as an antidote to the dialkyl-flurophosphates. (the nerve-gas)

Hyoscine is frequently used also as a preventive in sea and air motion sickness.

Hyoscyamine sulfate is used as sea sickness pills. Hyoscine is used also in obstetries, with morphine, as an analgesic agent to produce "twilight". sleep". It is also used as "truth-obtaining drug". Slight changes in the structure of the alkaloids has a profound effect on their physiological action. Thus only one optical isomer of stropine (hyoscyamine) has mydriatic properties. How-ever both isomers seem to have an equal effect on the central nervous system. Removal of the N-methyl group as in nor-hyoscyamine reduces the mydriatic activity quite considerably.

The ester group is essential for activity, tropine being inactive. Many esters have been synthesized from tropine and the most active drugs were obtained, when the esterifying acid was an aromatic one containing an asymmetric center. Simple esters such as tropine acetate have low activity. The steric position of the OH group in tropine is important. The esters of pseudo-tropine (XIII) have very low activity.

The distribution of the alkaloids in common Indian species is as follows, with slight variations occurring within the different genotypes.

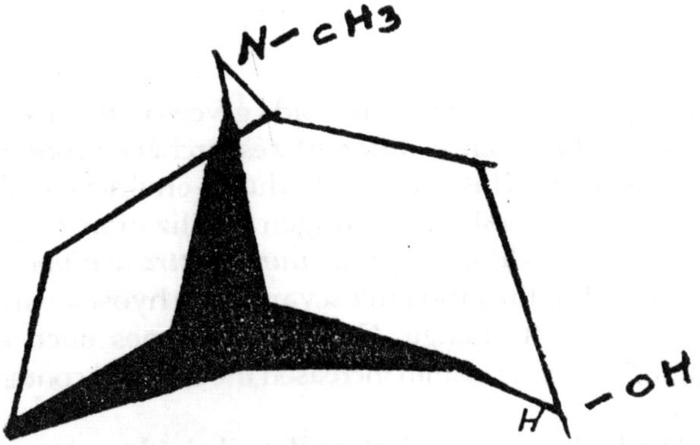

(XIII)

Species	Alkaloids	Authority
1. *D. metel* Linn.	Hyoscine-0.1 Hyoscyamine-0.4 Nor-hyoscyamine-0.1 Cusco-hygrine (in roots)-	Andrews[7], Guha[8b] Carr and Reynold[8] Jentzsch[9] Prasad.[10]
2. *D. innoxia* Mill.	Hyoscine-0.3 (total plant)-0.4 (in seeds)	Evans and partride[11]
	Hyoscyamine (with meteloidine) -0.6 (total-plant) 0.1 (in seeds)-	James[12] Steinegger and Gessler[13]
	Cuscohygrine (in roots) and an unknown alkaloid mp. 44-6C.	
	Hyoscyamine 0.4 (in leaves) 0.2 (in stams) 0.1 (in roots)	Andrews[7] Braun[15] Evans and Patride[16-17]
	Hyoscinne 0.1 (in leaves) 0.05 (in stem) 0.10 (in roots) 0.20 (in young plants)	Feldhaus[18]
	3,6-ditiglylteloidine (1001 roots) Cusco hygrine (in roots).	

The percentage weights of the alkaloids given on the above table, are average values. Since different researchers reported varying yield of alkaloids. This is probably due to environmental effects, races, genotypes, soil, etc. Nitrogen fertilization of the soil increase in alkaloid yield in *D. stramonium, D. stramonium, D. metel*, and *D. innoxia*, but the ratio f hyoscyamine to hyoscine in a particular species do not change. Growth hormones such as naphthoxyacetic acid, or zinc insulin increased the alkaloid content of *D. stramonium*.

Pruning[10] had a beneficial effect on the alkaloid-content of *D. stramonium* and *D. metel*. A short daily exposure of *D.strammonium* to ultra-violet light increased the alkaloid content.

The alkaloid content of D. stramonium was less after clear weather.[20]

A daily variation[21] was also found to occur in the alkaloids of this species, decreasing during the day and increasing at night. The alkaloid content of the seeds increased rapidly during the ripening process.

If the ripening was accelerated by exposure to carbon monoxide or acetylene the alkaloid contents of the seeds was less than normal.[20,22] When seeds of *D. stramonium* were exposed to X-rays and then germinated the plants were obtained with obvious morphological changes[24] but the nature and amount of the alkaloids was not significantly changed. However, Mothes and Co-Workers[25] have obtained mutants of *D. stramonium* which contain tobacco alkaloid, nicotine. The tetraploid races[24] of *Datura* have in general a slightly higher alkaloid percentage than the diploid races. The external factors like altitude, also influence alkaloid contents within the same species[26]. Using modern techniques, new alkaloids have been recorded in *Datura* genus.

Biogenesis of Datura Alkaloids

The sites of alkaloid synthesis in *Datura* vary with the species. In D. stramonium, the alkaloids are produced in the roots. This fact came to be known when hyoscyamine and hyoscine was produced in sterile root cultures of the plant[27]. Furthermore, a reduction in alkaloid content occurred when a *D. stramonium* scion was grafted onto an alkaloid-free root-stock such as tomato[28]

Alkaloids were detected in the roots shortly after germination of the seeds.[29]

Grafting experiments of *Atropa belladonna* with other species of Datura showed that leaves too are able to synthesize some of the tropane alkaloids[30]. Their experiments showed that hyoscine is produced mainly in the roots of *D. innoxia, D. metel* and *Atropa belladonna,* in the aerial parts of *D. meteloides* and in all parts of *D. ferox.,* while hyoscyamne is produced in all parts of *D. innoxia,* but mainly in the roots, meteloidine is produced only in the aerial parts of *D. ferox.*

Cuscohygrine[31] and 3,6-ditiglyteloidine have been detected only in the roots of Datura,[17] they are water-soluble and are conducted in transpiration stream, or in phloem, therefore location of this alkaloid dies not pin-point the site of synthesis. It is quite feasible that the basic skeleton of the alkaloid is synthesized in one part of the plant and N-methylation occurring in some other region. Quite less in known about the other metabolites occurring within the plant.

From the monumental work of Robinson[32,33,34,35], we record in-vitro synthesis of tropinone (XVII) as given by him.

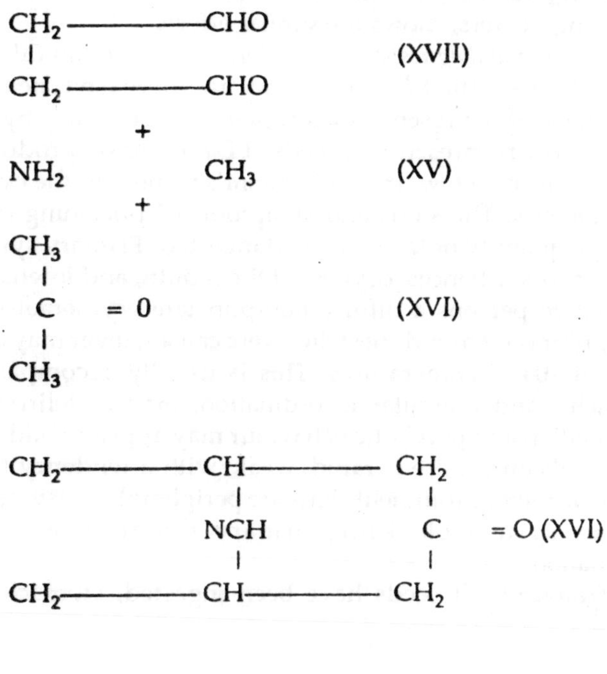

(XVII) (XV) (XVI) (XVI)

From succindi-aldehyde (XIV), methylamine (XV), and acetone (XVI) or acetone dicarboxylic acid. The reaction prevails within the plant.

The succindialdehyde get derived from Ornithine by oxidative deamination. The amino-acid, ornithine is produced from arginine by the action of the enzyme arginase.

Fuller and Gibson[36] noticed that the amount of this enzyme attain its peak in *D. stramonium*, when the production of alkaloid is at its maximum level.

Ornithine[37,38] is the precursor of the five membered ring of tropine (found by feeding radio-active ornithine). Putrescine is an intermediate between ornithine and succindiadehyde.[39]

Hyoscine on the other hand is derived from a different precursor, such as hydroxyornithine. Radio-active studies reveal that tropane ring is a derivative of tryptophane.[40]

The N-methyl-group of hyoscyamine is produced from methionine by transmethylation[41]. There is much more to be investigated before exact biogentic pathways for Daturalkaloids, could be clearly understood.

Toxicology : Ingestion of seeds of *Datura* causes atropine poisoning, further, intake of honey derived from atropine containing flowers, shows the similar effects.

Differential diagnosis : The patient records bilateral-dilation of pupils, dry flushed skin, and an increased heart rate. Confirmation of presence of atropine can be made by gastric lavage, showing presence of seeds of *Datura* or by production of mydriasis using a few drops of patient's urine into the eye of the cat. *Symptoms*: The signs and symptoms of poisoning depends upon the quantity of toxic material ingested. Primary symptoms are visual disturbances, dryness of the mouth, and intense thirst. In sensitive persons a diffuse non-punctate erythematous rash may appear on face and chest. In severe causes, fever may develop with 101-104°. Temperatures. This is usually accompanied by head-ache, and muscular incordination, mania, delirim visual hallucination and psychotic behaviour may appear, children may get convulsions. Pulse is rapid, weak, with a tendency towards dicrotism. Other prominent signs are peripheral parasympathetic nervous system blockade, urinary retention and severe constipation.

Treatment : If seeds have been ingested, stomach lavage

should be the first step. If parasympathetic blockade is present cholinergic drugs may be administered thereby relieving the dryness of mouth and tachycardia.[42]

Epilogue

The Art of healing in not new to Indians. As you have seen in the fore-going pages, Rig Vedas is a remarkable inventory of human knowledge, as old as third millennium B.C. (!). It records rhetorical description of Soma-plant which hitherto baffled the learned who stressed more on language origin rather than on scientific description. Had archaeologists and anthropologists cared to scrutinise the manifold sculptures and beautiful sculptured rockcaves of different era. Had these cared to look into the carved stones images of different tribes from Southern America, Siberia, etc., the picture would have been more clear, (cf. Plate.... Mushroom-Gods of Azetic Indians and Stone-rock of Kerala).

Indian school of Medicine (Ayurvedic system of Medicine) is a well organised system where-in the ailments of human body are well understood in mental, physiological, and physical planes.

The theory is that the five elements viz. prithvi, apas, vayu, jyoti and akasa constitute the human body. Life in its various manifestations originated as andaya, jarayuja and svedaja. The vayu (ether/wind) in the human organism is of five types according to physiological locations and functions. There are present parallel channels for 'Vayu' along with nervous system. These are interlinks between motor and sensory functions and even control of the seat of consciousness, with a control on the involuntary muscles.

Charaka[43] describes disease as an inequilibrium of "dhatus" (imbalance of forces of vayu) (Sut. IX. 1.4) Dhatus are made up of `Panchamahabhutas'[44]. When any external or internal forces come to play on human body "dhatus" get disturbed or unbalanced causing suffering or pain. When these `dhatus' are in "ucitapramana" (in proper flow and quantity) then body functions properly. "Dhatus" wax and wanes on particular hours of day and night (biological clock?) Disease or pain cause man to ingest drugs. Three drug-plants as used in Indian System of Medicine has been described.

In context to these drug-plants in question; very probably digestion of the properly filtered soma juice in mixture with milk brings about some change in fluid clectrolytes and acid-base balance in the human system which we now know is quite essential for saving life.

Man consume fluids and food which markedly vary both in quality and quantity, electrolyte levels of different individuals vary.

The organs which are constantly regulating the electrolyte levels are the intestine and the kidneys. The process by which they per form this useful function is termed as "internal circulation of salts". Principal extracellular ions enter the lumen of the G.I. tract and renal tubules and they in their turn regulate electrolyte levels (cf. Qurt. Med. Rev. 20 (3 & 4). 1970).

As already stated elsewhere above that soma juice is high diuretic, suggesting that it probably brings about electrolyte in balance; and kidneys trying to wash out the toxins (?). Further it is observed that it effects the central nervous system. Spinal cord, controls common reflexes, medulla oblongata the balancing postures, etc.; cerebellum, gravity impulses; cerebrum, with its hypothalamus controls thermostatic variations. The body heat produces through a constant gentle vibrations of the muscles from 7-13 times per second. Hypothalamus senses the temperature of blood passing through it and controls it.

It also detects water concentration in the blood and works through pituitary gland to adjust the work of the kidneys. Hypothalamus measures the sugar concentration in the blood, and sets up hunger sensations. Thus the body mechanism is intricately interconnected with the hypothalamus. Upper parts of Cerebrum controls conscious motion and sensations. The brain contain cells rich in ribonucleic acid (RNA). These cells have a capacity of varying slightly in structure producing trillions of delicately different varieties of RNA. RNA controls construction of protein molecules within the cell and each different RNA molecule can bring about the manufacture of a slight different protein molecule. A little change in RNA molecules therefore changes the protein molecule structure. This effects the memory probably sap of Soma brings much greater change within the brain cell nuclei. The mushrooms contain a series of toxic amino-acids and alkaloids which undergoes some change which causes change of the brain cells to thus bringing about rejuvenation of the human system.

According to Chinese Internal Medical classic " of Nei Ching (5th Century B.C.). The human body has 365 vital points (*Hsuch Tao*) which on being punched by a needle release" bad secretion or gas and relieves the tissues concerned of their obstructions. Each of these points are duly termed and assigned functions with the internal organs and also with the circulatory system. This type of therapy is practised by Indians and Chinese who und- -stood the concepts of the disease and their "vital links" along the circulatory system. The Chinese system of Medicine, believes in a theory of double circulation by which the `*spirits* or gaes (Vayu) are vehicles round the *Yon principles* (-) and the blood which conveys the *Yang* principle (+). These are distributed throughout the body. According to it the circulation begins in the lungs at 3'O clock in the morning at the hour of Tiger and completes its rounds within 24 hours. The circulation is carried through twelve principal channels (chin), six of them flow head downwards, while the remaining six from leg-upwards. There are in addition accessory canals, eight of which run transversely and nine obliquely.

There are in addition three main "burning spaces" ("Agni kunda") which serve as a exhaust channels from the twelve canals into the internal bladder, and which also serves a s a storage space for *yin* (–) and (+) principles. According to Chinese medical school, these are two most important opposing forces. Everything in the universe including heath is dependent upon the balances of these forces (dhatus). They designate these as + or –, male or female, ebb and flow, life and death, wet and dry, sun and moon, heat and cold, etc. By acupunctures one can get relief of gases (Vayu) obstructions, leading to the restoration of the Yin and Yang principles which however is much alike our Ayurvedic Principles, but explained in different terminology.

As regards *Cannabis*, it was only used by 'Yogis, who wish to attain perfection in controlling their internal secretion by yoga. It is linked with hormonal balance. Much in this direction is to be understood before anything positive could be said about it. It is known to bring about nervous disturbance if not properly used.

The third-plant *Datura*, which is also used for mental levation, effects the nervous and the digestive system if not properly used.

It is now clear that all the three drug-plants effects the Central nervous system and digestive tracts; a thorough study should be made of the "internal circulation of Vayu" it channels and orifies.* It has definite link with nervous system. It would not out of way to mention that "acupuncture"** techniques which is being followed in Chinese system of Medicine*** also record presence of gas or nerve channels which when punched or blocked gives relief to disordered organs. In Hindu religious ceremonies, generally the lobes of ears are punched. This has now found to be useful in the cure of bronchial diseases especially the asthma.

In conclusion, it may be pointed out that the older authentic Rig Vedic texts should be carefully scrutinized and interpretated for proper and judicious use of these famous Indian Drugs.

References

1. Karnick, C.R. and MD. Saxena: *Datura* Linn, the famous narcotic from the East. —A review Quart. J. Crude, Drug, Res. (Netherlands) 10 (1): 1493-1516 (1970).
2. Cooper, J.M: Stimulants and narcotics. The comparative Ethnology of South American Indians. Smithsonian Instit. Bull. No. 143 5: 525-558 (1949).
3. Saxena, MD.: Genus *Datura* Linn. Ph.D. thesis Vikram University Ujjain (1971).
4. Henry, T.A: The plant alkaloids 4th ed. Churchill, Ltd. London, 804 pp. (1949).
5. Holmes, H.L: The chemistry of tropane alkaloids. In Mansks and Homles (eds). The alkaloids. I: 271-374.
6. Foder, G: Recent development in the synthesis and stereochemistry of tropane alkaloids. Tetrahedron 1: 86-102 (1957).
7. Andrews, A.E.: The active constituents of the Indian Solanaceous plant. Datura stramonium *D. fastuosa* and *D. metel*. Jour. Chem. Soc. (London) *99*: 1871-1877. (1911).

---

* There are nine internal (Vayu) orifices, for gaseous exchange. (cf. Shastri H. 1971. Jour Res. Indian Med. 5(2), 183).

** Albert Field (1947): Ancient Chinese Surgery : Acupuncture Calif. Med. 67 : 39-40.

*** According to Yoga concepts, there are three principles nerves namely the *ida*, the *pingala* and the *Susumna*. These originate around the waist on and runs along the vertebral column into the skull to the fore-head. The *ida* and pingala coalase to form an outer loop encasing the *susumna* in the centre, where they converge, the point is termed as 'untied triple junction,' this point of confluence is situated at the fore-head between the eyebrows and is known as "the liberated triple junction", Deep concentration of mind leads to be activation of "*Susumna* (while ida and pingala becomes insert) leading to enlightenment. How the above mentioned drugs effects these nerve centres is yet to be known to modern medical science.

8. Carr, F.H. and Reynolds, W.C: Nor-hyoscyamine and nor-atropine; alkaloids, occurring in various Sojanaceous plants. Trans. Chem. Soc. (London) 101kg 946-958 (1912).

8b. Guha, MP.: The alkaloid content of *Datura metal*. *Indian Pharmacist* 6: 201-206 (1951)(.

9. Jentzsch, K: Contribution to the knowledge of alkaloid formation in Solanaceous plants. *Sci*. Pharmaceut 21: 285-291 (1953).

10. Prasad, S: Effects of pruning and exploration on the growth and alkaloid content of *Datura metal* L. J. Am. Pharm. Sci. Ed. 37 : 346-349 (1948).

11a. Evans, W.C. and M.W. Partridge: Alkaloid biogenesis part I: the site of synthesis of alkaloids in *Datura*. Jour. Pharm. and Pharmacol. 5: 293-300 (1953a)

11b. Evans, W.C. and M.W. Partridge: Alkaloid biogensis Part KK. Changes in the ontogenetic production of alkaloids in *Atropa* and *Datura*. Jour. Pharm. and Pharmcol. 5: 772-777 (1953b).

12. James, W.O: Alkaloid formation in plants. Jour. Pharm. and Pharmacol. 5: 809-822 (1953).

13. Steinegger, E and f. Gessler: Alkaloidal biogenesis in *Datura innoxia*. Pharm. Acta Helv. 30: 115-123 (1955).

14. Gerlach. W.O: *Datura innoxia*—a potential commercial sources of scopolamine. Economic Bot. 2 : 436-454 (1948).

15. Braum, W: The influence of long-wave ultra-violet radiation on the constituents of different drug-plants. Beitr. Biol. Pflanz. 26: 331-400 (1939).

16. Evans, W.C. and M.W. patridge: Alkaloid of *Datura innoxia* Nature: 171: 656. (1953c).

17. Evans, W.C. and M.W. Partridge: 7-hydroxy-3.6 ditigly-loxytropane, a new alkaloid isolated from the roots of *Datura*. Jour. Chem. Soc. 1102-113 (1957).

18. Feldhaus, J: Quantitative estimation of the distribution of the alkaloids in the various parts of *D. stramonium* L. Arch. Pharm. 243, 328-348 (1905).

19. Guillon, A: The alkaloids of *Datura stramonium* and the course of their development. *Compt. Rendu* 230: 1604-1606 (1950).

20. Hegnauer, R: The influence of external factors on the content of active compounds in medicinal plants IV. The daily fluctuations of the alkaloid content in the leaves of *Atorpa, Atura* and Hyoscyamus. Pharm. Weekblad. 88: 106-112 (1953).

21. Hemberg, I and H. Fluck: The daily periodicity of the content of alkaloids and other nitrogen-containing substances in *D. stramonium*-Pharm. Acta. Helv. 28: 74-85 (1953).

22. Johnson, C.H. and E. Nunez-Melendez: A study of wild and cultivated stramonium in Puerto. Reo. J. Amer. Pharm. Assoc. *31* : 166-169 (1942).

23. Otsuka, K. and T. Nagata: Effect of nitrogen levels on the alkaloid content of medicinal plants with special references to Datura stramonium, J. Sci. Soil. Manure (Japan): 24: 149-152 (1953).

24. Rowson, J.M.: Increased alkaloidal contents of induced polyploids of Datura, Atropa and Hyoscyamus Part I: Datura species. Quart. J-Pharm. Pharmacol. 18: 175-184 (1945).

25. Mothes, K: A Romoeike, and H.B. Schroter: Mutation experiments with alkaloid producing plants Die. Naturwissenschaften 42: 214 (1955).

26. Karnick, C.R. and M.D. Saxena, On the variability of alkaloid production in *Datura* species. *Planta Medica* 18 (1970).

27. Stinstra, T.M.: Formation of mydriatic alkaloids in excised root-cultures of *D. stramonium* grown on a completely synthetic nutrient. Proc: Moningkl. Ned. Akad. Wetenschap. 57c.: 584-593 (1954).
28. Jackson, B.P. and Rowson, J.M.: Alkaloid biogenesis in tetraploid stramonium. Jour. Pharm. and Pharmacol. 5: 778-793 (1950).
29. Guillon, A: The alkaloids of *Datura stramonium* and the course of their development. Compt. Rendu 230:1604-1606 (1950).
30. Shibata, S. and Imaseki I: Phytochemical investigation on cultivation of Medicinal plants VIII. On alkaloid biogenesis in Datura. J. Pharm. Soc. (Japan) 74: 862-865 (1954).
31. Haga, P.P. Van: Cuscohygrine, a normal constituent alkaloid of Atropa belladonna. Nature 174: 833-834 (1954).
32. Robinson, R: A Synthesis of tropinone. J. Chem. Soc. 3: 762-763 (1917).
33. Robinson, R: Theory of the mechanism of the phyto-chemical synthesis of certain alkaloids. J. Chem. Soc. 3 : 876-899 (1917).
34. Robinson, R: Synthesis in Biochemistry, J. Chem. Soc. 1079-1090 (1936).
35. Robinson, R: The structural relations of natural products. Oxford, C: Arendon Press. (1955).
36. Fuller W.C. and M.R. Gibson. The arginase-alkaloid relationship in *D. tatula (D. stramonium)* Jour. Amer. Pharm. Assoc. 41: 263-266 (1952).
37. Leete, E: Lamarion and I.D. Spenser, Biogenesis of hyoscyamine. Nature *174*: 650-651 (1954a).
38. Leete, E: L. Marion, and I.D. Spenser: The biogenesis of alkaloids. XII. The mode of formation of tropine base of hyoscyamine, Can. J. Chem, 32: 1116-1123 (1954b).
39. Cromwell, B.T.: Studies on the synthesis of hyoscyamine in Atropa Belladonna and Datura stramonium L. Bio. Chem. J. 37 : 717-722 (1944a).
Cromwell, B.T.: The role of putrescine in the synthesis of hyoscyamine. Biochem. J. 37 : 722-726 (1944).
40. Mortimer, P.I: A Possible common biogenetic origin of the nicotine, torpane, and hygrine bases. Nature 172: 74-75 (1953).
41. Marion, L and A. F. Thomas: A further observation on the biogenesis of hyoscyamine. Cam. J. Chem. 33: 1853-1854 (1955).
42. Lamps, K.F. and Rune Fagerstrom; Plant toxicity and Dermatits: The Williams and Wilkins Co. Baltimore (1968).
43. Charaka Samhita: Agnivesha Nirnaya Sagar Press. Bombay (1941).
44. Gupta L.P: (1967) Concepts of diseases and its relation with doses. Surruta Ayurveda, 137-151.

VI

DATURA LINN

The Famous Narcotic of the East

Introduction

The plant *Datura* has been used as a narcotic, in India, since time immemorial. In old Indians literature it is referred to as 'Shivashekhara' since the flowers and fruits were said to be blessed by Lord Siva an Indian deity; for attaining mental peace.

The word *Datura* is derived from the sanskrit word "Dhatura" which generally refers to the capsules of *D. metel*.

Blakeslee[4] has done a monumental work on the genetical aspect of the aspect of the genus *Datura*. He has contributed much to our knowledge of heredity and has proved that even a study of a single plant in varied aspects of biology could reveal much to our existing knowledge. The frontiers of knowledge are continuously changing i.e., they are dynamic and therefore, one finds new additions to pre-existing facts. Much has been done by Blakeslee and his associates[4] but still much more is to be done. The present paper attempts reviewing all facets of observations on *Datura* plant which has not been complied after 1959.

The subject matter has been critically analysed under different headings. These are as follows:

Morphology

Wein Kurt give an historical account of *Datura stramonium* while parclay[7] outlines a new systematic position to the various species of *Datura*. He suggests *D. meteloides* DC ex Dunal, be termed as D. innoxia Mill, since he says they are identical in every morphological character.

Linsley[100] studied the pollination of *Datura* species growing wild in Mexican deserts. Flowers were found to be visited by matinal bees.

Maniquis[110] made some comparative studies on *D. metel* and *D. meteloides* and found some diagnostic differences between them.

Fosberg[51] brought to light some of the nomenclature differences of different species of *Datura.*

Reifman[130] observed in developmental studies of the flower of *D. fastuosa* that the calyx was transformed into corolla. This transformation of floral brought in doubling of corolla.

Gerasimenko[54] studied the intra-specific variation in *D. innoxia*. He was able to differentiate on the basis of morphological and physiological differences, four newforms which he identifies as f-*vulgaris*, f-*microcrapa*, f-*robusta* and f-*longquipedunculata*. He records that the forms -*vulquaris* of *D. innoxia* produced highest percentage of alkaloids in comparison with other forms.

Skogen[156] records presence of *D. stramonium* from Trondheim regions of Norway.

Madal et al screened some of the Indian species and varieties of *Datura* plants for *alkaloids*.

Yankoulov studied the phylogensis of the genus *Datura.*

Ismailov[69] made some ecological and floristic analysis on the *Datura* species found in Talysk.

Pratsap Singh and Kaul[128] found that polyploids varieties of the *D. innoxia* showed higher percentage of alkaloids than the controls.

Jain[70] records D. innoxia growing well in inhospitable regions of Rajasthan Desert (India).

Lynn[106] noticed D. stramonium growing in some parts of North Ireland.

Sandberg[135] records species of *Datura* from places in Ecuador, Peru and Chili.

Bristol[13] noticed tree species growing in Hawaii Islands. These were Datura sanquinea; *D. candida* and *D. suaveolens*.

Seed Germination

Soriano et al[165] studies the factors governing the processes in the germination of *D. ferox* and found that the germination of seeds is blocked immediately after ripeness, by an inhibitor. Removal of seed coat and certain storage conditions promotes germination by either diffusion of the inhibitor or its destruction. On removal of inhibitor they become positively photoblastic, responding to R-FR mechanism. Another interesting fact brought out by their study was the effect of red light could be replaced by gibberellic acid treatment.

Sanchez et al[136] in their studies on seed germination of *Datura ferox* found that gibberellic acid (GA) eliminated the germination blockage in photoblastic *D. ferox* seeds. They also noticed that maximum response to GA was found with wetted decoated dormant seeds. This indicates certain metabolic processes should take place before GA can effect. These processes are reduced or at much slower rate if seed coats are intact.

Gugliada et al[61] investigated the relationship of seed coat to photo-induction in germination of *D. ferox* seeds. They found that in decoated photoblastic *Datura ferox* seeds, the length of the incubation period which proceeds irradiation with red light affects their response to this treatment. Although the behaviour of the intact seeds shows the same tendency, the germination counts do not reach the same values. These differences between the intact and decoated seeds decrease as after ripening advances. The presence of seed coat during the incubation period which precedes irradiation brings about a situation which can depending on the stage of after ripening, advances the light requirements for maximum response decreases as does the level of inhibitor present in the seeds. The physiological situation may be due to the effect of oxidative processes within the seeds.

Pozeulo and Razario de Pelipe[126] outlines a rapid method of germination *D. stramonium* seeds.

Gerasimenko[54] studied some aspects of seed germination of D. innoxia and found that the temperature plays a significant role in its germination.

Jankulov[72] studied the relationships between germination percentage and the available quantity of water, in the seeds of *D. stramonium, D. fastuosa* and *D. tatual*. He found that seeds of *Datura* varieties react specifically to increased water content. Most sensitive to an increased water supply were *D. metel, D. meteloides* and *D. stramonium*. Resistant species were found to be *D. innermis, D. ceratocaula,* and *D. innoxia*. His findings could be useful for the evaluation of a suitable variety for plantation in a given locality.

Cultivation

Caesar[17] records various methods of cultivations of *D. stramonium* and *D. metel* used by him in Germany.

Fertilizers

El-Hamidi et al[36] observed the effect of chemical fertilizers on the growth, yield and alkaloid production in *D. stramonium* var. *innermis* grown in U.A.R. They found that plants subjected to different levels of N.P.K., with addition of N. leads to an increase of number and dry weight of leaves. N_4 level increased the dry weight by 15 percent, over the control, while the combination of N. and P. leads to slight increase, NPK leads to increase in height and dry weights of stems and roots. Addition of N. results an increase of dry weight of pericaps and seeds. Also it results in increase of total alkaloids.

Sinja and Verma[158] studied the effect of fertilizer on the growth and alkaloid contents of *Datura innoxia*. They found that plants treated with potassium nitrate (KNO_3) yielded a significant higher dry weight and alkaloidal content per plant as compared to controls.

Diseases

Hirst and Moore[66] in their study on new plant diseases and pests records *Datura* plant being infected by phytophthera *infestens*.

Morgan[116] records leaf curl disease attacking *D. stramonium*.

Singh and Mathur[159] records infection of *Cercospora daturicola* (Sepg.) Vassiljevsky on *Datura stramonium*.

Hildebrand et al[65] in their investigations on bacterial enhancement of self limiting out growth formation on *Datura* found that the differences in size and stability of out growths formed in association with pseudomonas were due in part to invivo indole-acetic-acid production by the pathogen.

Lovrekovich and Loebenstein[101] were able to induce nonhyperplastic galls on *D. stramonium* leaves by living and heat-killed phytopathogenic bacteria namely *Pseudomonans* syrinqae, *P. Lachrymans* and *P. phaseolicola*.

Force[50] investigated the mechanism of selection by phytophagons insects, some species of plants for their survival.

He found that neither the larvae nor the adults responded to synthetic nutrient and non-nutrient diets containing *Datura* leaf extract or leaf powders. All evidence indicated that the feeding behaviour of the insect is conditioned by a combination of factors in the food medium.

Manigault and Beaud[112] found that the tumors could be induced in the tissues of stems of *D. Stramonium* by inoculation with *Aqrobacterium tumifacieus*.

Dimitri-Jevic[35] was able to reactivate sporulation of *Alternaria crassa* with the held of leaves of *Datura* species. Sterile mycelium sown on leaves begins to produce conidia after 5 to 7 days at room temperature. The virulence of this isolate is also reactivated for use in inoculation.

Manigault and Beaud[111] studied the phyto-pathogenic properties of different strains of *Agrobacterium tumefacieus* on *D. stramonium*.

Virus

Blattney et al[10] noticed that big virus could be induced in *D. stramonium* plants.

Quantz[129] records a ring spot virus infecting *D. stramonium* plants.

Shorin et al[155] noticed that the upper surface of the leaves of *D. stramonium, D. alba* and *D. bernherdi* was easily infected with TM virus.

Ghiu, Ren-Jong and Sill[23] found that *D. stramonium* was suitable host for brome-gras mosaic virus. It can flourish well.

They[22] also studied the factors effecting the control of brome-grass mosaic virus on *Datura stramonium*. Loebenstein and frankross[102] found that extracts obtained from *D. strasmonium* plants could induce infection of tobacco mosaic virus.

Lukasiak[105] studied pecten methyl esterase activities in healthy and tumerus (agro-bacterium infected) stem tissue of *D. stramonium*. He found that pecten-methylesterase (PME) activity was comparatively higher in tumors than in the stem tissues and in two moths old tumours it was about 2 to 5 times.

Summanwar and Hooker[163] studied the cytopathology of the potato virus during different growth stages of the cotyledons of *D. tatula*.

Verma and Verma records mosaic virus effecting *D. metel* leaf.

Kardos[80] was able to isolate a micro organism from *D. stramonium* seeds. He found that micro-organism and the seed contained the same pigment. He noticed qualitative and quantitative similarity between the amino acids of *Datura* seeds and those of micro-organism. Immunological investigations (agglutination, precipitation tests) revealed a marked similarity between the immunological properties of proteins isolated from *Datura* seeds and the micro-organism. The micro-organism contained a factor which exhibited a pharmological and biological atropine reaction. The factor isolated in crystalline form induced an atropine like reaction in the eye of the cat. Results shown that a new form of symbiosis occur between the plant cell and micro-organism.

Carroll et al[18] records findings in local lesions of *D. stramonium* presence of tobacco mossaic virus.

Summanwar[162] studied the cytopathology of potato virus in cotyledons of D. tatula under different stages of growth.

Cohen and Nitzany[26] investigated the presence of tomato yellow leaf curl virus (Bemisia tabaci) on *D. stramonium*.

Zhuk and Kishko[190] studied the localization and gradual spread of X-virus antigen of potatoes into the tissue of *D. stramonium*. The virus antigen was found on the third day after infection in the primarily infected epidermis and parenchyma of the conducting bundles.

Carroll and Shalla[18] noticed the lesion development and the distribution of tobacco mosaic virus in the D. stramonium. He found that when leaves of *D. stramonium* were inoculated with a common strain of tobacco mosaic virus, narcotic local lesions developed after 3 days, while after seven days the lesions consisted of three distinct color zones. Many lesions increased in size until the leaf became seniscent and abscised in about 40 days. Ineffectively infectivity. He found that transmission was easier in young seedlings of *D. innoxia* and *D. tatual*.

Eskarous[48] records a new distortion strain of tobacco mosaic virus infecting local lesions of *Datura stramonium*.

Kahn[78] isolated a new virus of potato virus Y group from *Datura candida* and *D. sanquinea* imported from Sibundoy valley, Putumayo, Colombia.

Kaul[84] noticed that when *D. quercifolia* was infected with mosaic virus there was a complete breakdown of the emiotic process, chiefly synapsis at diakinesis and at metaphase. As a result the presence of univalents caused many irregularities in the later stages of meiosis. There was a significant reduction of pollen fertility and the mean number of seeds per capsule.

Herbicides

Fites, slife and Hanson[49] fed *D. stramonium* with carboxyl-labelled C^{14} 2,4-dichlorophenoxyacetic acid (2, 4-D). Autoradiographs and extractions of radioactive materials showed the path followed by the herbicide. It was found that the activity decreased in the leafy tissues while there was an accumulation of activity within the stems and little accumulation in roots. There was a total loss of radioactivity in the root systems which indicated possible detoxification mechanism in *D. stramonium*. Twenty-five percent of 2,4-D applied to Datura was expelled from roots within six weeks time.

Bailey[6] records the weeding out of *Datura ferox* and *D. stramonium* a common pest in grain fields of Queensland by 2,4-D amine.

Eshel[41] studied the effects of herbicide BV-207 on Datura plants. He found BV-207 was toxic to plants. It interferes with photosynthesis and inhibits root growth.

Cytology

Singh and Fatima[160] noticed that several plants of *D. metel* showed a wide range of morphological variations and cytological irregularities particularly in the number and behaviour of chromosomes. All stages of meiotic division were found in the same anther in basipetal succession. A single large nucleolus was observed in first prophase. In addition to the normal 12 bivalents, 24 bivalents were observed in about 6.12 percent of the microsporocytes. Chiasma frequency and terminalization co-efficient in both diploid and teraploid cells was determined. A complete or partial failure of chromosome pairing was observed. Of a total of 24 chromosomes asynapis occurred in 2 to 18 chromosomes and sometimes all the 24 chromosomes failed to pair. These univalents generally divide into two chromatids at anaphase and then distribution becomes normal.

Genetics

Little[99] studied gene segregation in auto-tetraploids of some species of *Datura*.

Romeike[132] in his investigations on *Datura* hybrids, found that *D. ferox* has an ability to convert hyoscyamine into hyoscine, but it depends upon its heredity. In as much he found that hybrids of *D. ferox* and *D. stramonium* in F_1 generation are typically hyoscine plants, more over they showed heterosis effect in growth. By selection of generation he was able to obtain F_4 generation belonging uniformly to the hyoscine type. In some cases there was uniformity in growth between the descendent of individuals of F_3 generation. There sizes were favourable as that of F_1 generation but their fertility was very unsatisfactory. Further he treated seeds of hybrids obtained from *D. ferox* and D. stramonium with colchicine and could produce a tetraploid in C generation (corresponding to the F_1 generation of diploid hybrids). This generation were typical hyocine plants but anthocyanine content of the plants were not uniform.

Trudgill et al noticed the effect of resistant solanaceous plants on the sex ratio of *Heterodera rostochiensis* and the use of the sex ratio to assess the frequency and genetic constitution to the pathophytes. They found larvae could not survive on the roots of *Datura stramonium*.

Anatomy

Walker studied the effect of mechanical stimulation on the collenchyma tissue of the plants of *D. stramonium*. He found that such stimulation greatly increased the amount of wall-thickening per cell, but it inhibits cell elongation. When plants were subjected to mechanical stimulus in darkness, the collenchymatous tissue showed reduction in wall thickening and he suggests that reduction of wall material was due to its utilization as substrate for respiratory processes which occurred in the plant under such abnormal condition.

Akisue Gokithi[1] noticed some anatomical variation in samples of *D. stramonium* obtained from two different regions of the city of Sao Paulo. One sample obtained from North west the other from South West region of the City. Leaves of the plant obtained from the North west showed numerous crystals, sand idioblasts containing large tertrahydric crystals in the ribs while plants from South West were devoid of these features.

Pharmacognosy

Dechyshyn[28] records some microscopic diagnosis of the fruit and seeds of D. innoxia. According to him, *D. innoxia* fruits are distinguished by the presence of a large number of filaments on a multicellular pedicel of a single celled head and longitudinal folds of cuticle on the outer epidermis. The seeds of *D. innoxia* are characterized by thickened out epidermis with lenticular thickening on the lateral walls of the cells.

Shah and Khanna[148] carried out pharmacognostic studies of the stem and leaf of *D. metel* and *D. metel* var *fastuosa*. They record some structural differences between the two species.

Tissue-Culture

Gross a nd Shutte[63] in their experimentation with D. Metal root tissue cultures observed that phenylalamine 3-C^{14}) could be used as a component for the synthesis of the tropic acid in hyoscyamine and scopolamine. They found that bezoic acid could be successfully used for the synthesis of cocaine by rooted twings of *Erythroxylum novogranatense*. After hydrolysis of alkaloids and oxidative degeneration of tropic acid, the total activity could be shown to be, in the benzoic acid, this shows the direct incorporation of phenylalamine to tropic and benzoic acids.

Sullivan and Gibson[161] experimented on the root cultures of *D. stramonium* Linn var tatula Tor. and *D. innoxia* Mill found that when proline C^{14} was made available to roots, it was incorporated into hyoscyamine and scopolamine, and at the same time the root growth was effected in both species.

Guha and Mahesuari[160] records in-vitro production of embroys from the anthers of *Dautra*. They were able to produce embryos which developed into normal seedlings. Most of the-embryos appeared to be located inside the pollensacs and were free floating. They suggests that they may have arisen from the pollen grains or from the connected tissues of the anthers.

Chan, Wen-Nuei and Staba[21] in their tissue culture studies in Dautra callus, records that they found alkaloid content varied from 0.004% in *D. stramonium* tetraploid stem callus to 0.056% in *D. innoxia* seed callus. Seed callus of *D. stramonium* and *D. innoxia* contain more alkaloids (0.016-0.056%) that root (0.012-0.015%) stem (0.004-0.014%) or leaf callus (0.010-0.007%). The highest Datura alkaloid production (1.4 mg/gm dry weight tissue) was obtained from 3-weeks old tissue. The tissue had been grown in MT-1 medium for two and in MT-1 medium with a L-ornithine-HCL (0.2%) and L. Phynylalamine (0.2%)mixture for additional week. Thin layer chromatogram indicated that the hyoscine is the principal alkaloid in suspension cells grown in MT-1 medium with yeast extract (0.2%) Hyoscine has been reported to be the major alkaloid present in aseptic root of *Datura*.

Elze and Teusher[39] experimented on the uptake and storage of alkaloids in the tissue cultures of *Datura* species, and found that submerged grown single cells of Datura species were able to take up added atropine from the medium and to accumulate it. The levels reached in the mediums were much higher than the concentration of alkaloids in the surrounding solution. The accumulation is inhibited by 2, 4-dinitrophenol and sodium azide. Application of other alkaloids (scopolamine, chimine, lokeline, codeine, papaverine, pilocarpine and yohimbine) showed specificity of the reaction. They assume that the protoplast is an active participant in the accumulation process.

Jindra and Staba[76] investigated the Datura tissue cultures and found that in cultures arginase, transminage and esterase activities were present but when arginine, ornithine, phenylalamine, tropine and tropic acid were used as substrate, specific reaction were noticed. Furthermore they[166a] noticed in tissue cultures obtained from chlorophilous and non-chlorophilous strains that maganese (14 ppm). stimulated the production of cuscolygine, choline, and pseudotropine. Aminoacid precursors or chlorophillous tissue had no significant effect upon the production of these alkaloids. Hyoscyamine or scopolamine were not detectable.

Physiology

Massini[114] found that photosynthetic phosphorylation could be an explanation for induction phenomenon in photo-synthesis of Datura leaves.

Walker records the change brought about on collenchyma of *D. stramonium* by mechanical stimulation and etiolation.

Karkoszka et al[81] noted the effects3 of acclimatization on *D. innoxia*. They found that during growth of plant the highest percentage of alkaloids were found in the roots (0.26-0.30%) and in unripe seeded capsules (0.41%). On reaching maturity the seeds showed (0.24-0.46%) stems 0.10%) and leaves (0.6-0.10%). Leaves showed lower percentage of alkaloid in comparison to flowering tops of the shoots. (0.10-0.23%).

Wassberg investigated the effects of 2,4-D on the flowers and fruits of *D. stramonium* and *D. tatula*.

Brucker and Schmidt[16] studied the sugar metabolism of callus and crown gall tissue of *Datura*. They report 30-50% higher than that of callus tissue. Fermentation activity is smaller but is 30% higher for tumor than for callus tissue. Metabolic activity appears not to be related to growth rate. None of the acids of Kreo's cycle accumulates in these cultures. Their content is some what lower in crown gall than incallus tissue.

Effects of inhibitors showed no difference between the two types of tissue in glyclysis, the pentose-phosphate cycle or in the effect of sulfhydryl blocks or heavy metal complex formation. Inhibition of the tricarboxylic acid cycle by flueroacetic and malonic acid and uncoupling of oxidative phosphoxylation by 2,4-dinitrophenol required high concentration in tumour than in callus tissue. Final oxidation in callus seems to depend more on the cytochrome system that of tumour tissue on the ascorbib acid system.

Kolodziejski and kulesyna[90] investigated the localization of tropine alkaloids in *D. stramonium* during development. The found that the highest content was observed during full blooming, in leaves upto 0.50% and in stems upto 0.36%.

Evans and Griffin[42, 43] in their observations on the production of alkaloids in the roots of *D. innoxia* under various conditions in cultures, found that the best yield of alkaloids was in roots (0.19% dry weight grown in sand cultures). Ditigloyl esters of dihydroxytropanes was (0.07%) in herbs grown in sand cultures.

Shpilenya[157] studied the effect of insufficient moisture of the soil on the alkaloid accumulation in genus *Datura*. He found that the presence of insufficient moisture in the soil had a negative effect on the growth and formation of reproductive organs of *D. inermis* and *D. stramonium*. Further he found that decreased percentage of moisture in the soil changes in the dynamics of alkaloid accumulation within the plant during initial stages. Dry conditions bring about the increase in the percentage contents of alkaloids while prolonged dryness in the soils brings about decrease in alkaloid percentage.

Sciuchetti[139] experimented on *D. meteloides* and noted the influence on kinetin and gibbrellic acid on the growth and alkaloid patterns. He found significant increase in the height of the plants when they were treated with GA. where as those treated with kinetin were shorter in height, than controls. Considerable decrease in dry weights were noted in GA treated plants, while reduction were observed in kinetin treated plants. The concentration of alkaloids in the organs of the plants treated with GA markedly reduced but insignificant change occurred within those treated with kinetin. The total alkaloid content per plant was less in each of the treated groups but total stem alkaloids was much greater in those treated with G.A. It was also noticed that percentage of chlorophyll a and b decreased with GA, but increased with kinetin treatment.

Vagujfalvi investigated the mineral nutrition of *D. innoxia*.

Evans and Griffin[43] noticed that, diligloyt esters of hydroxy tropanes are usually found in the roots of *Datura* spp. It also occurs in the transpiration stream of *D. innoxia* and D. cornigera, although they do not accumulate the products in the aerial parts. They therefore, suggest that an alkaloid previously isolated from the roots or leaves of a number of species and now recorded from the transpiration stream is probably an optical somer of nor-hyoscine. Hyoscine was the principal alkaloid of the sap of both the species investigated at the same time, noratropine and norhyoscine were also present.

Gibson and French[56] studied the effect of gibberelic acid on the growth and alkaloid synthesis in *Datura Stramonium* var tatual root cultures. They found that in low concentration of gibberellic acid (10,20,60 ppm.) the root showed inhibition in growth, development of filamentious adventitious roots and a low alkalloid content as compared to controls, while an increase in gibberellic acid percentage to 60 ppm., brought about higher increase in alkaloid content.

Gibson and Abbott[55] investigated the effect of proline on growth and alkaloid synthesis in *D. stramonium* root cultures. They found that exogenous proline effects the metabolism within the species.

Caldwell and Sciuchetti[25] recorded the effect of gibberellin and other treatments on the germination and subsequent biogenesis of alkaloids in *Datura stramonium*. They found that when seeds were subjected to cold treatments, the rate and germination percentage was reduced, whereas when they were treated with Gibberellin (GA) and concentrated H_2SO_4 (SA) the germination percentage increased. Plants growth with G.A. treatments showed fluctuation in the alkaloid concentration in different organs at different stages of growth.

Bennet and Sciuchetti[8] investigated the effects of various growth regulators on Datura meteloides and found that when it was treated with Amox-1618, concentration of alkaloids increased by 26% in roots while those treated with AMAB phosphon showed increase by 17%. The total alkaloid content was increased by 25% in leaf tops of plants treated with CO-11, 32% in roots treated with Amox-1618. There was marked increase of about 18% in chlorophyll concentration in plants treated phosphon, B 995 and CO-11 groups.

James and Sciuchetti[71] studied the action and interaction of gibberellic acid and B995 on *D. innoxia*. They found that gibberellic acid (GA) treated plants increased in height but showed decreased alkaloid concentration. Similar results were seen in plants treated with B995.

Sciuchetti and Mingis[141] noticed the effect of dimethyl sulfoxide (DMSO) and tributyl 2, 4-dichlorobenzlphosphonium chloride (Phosphon) on the growth and alkaloid synthesis in Datura ferox. They found the plant was simulated in growth by DMSO and which increases the total alkaloid production. Phosphon caused 43% reduction in plant height and 61% in total plant weight, with significant reduction in total alkaloid content per plant, but showed 33% increase in the concentration of the stem and root alkaloids. Phosphon was found to be a growth inhibitor not a growth retardant.

Erasmus[47] investigated the delayed incompatibility in the graft combination of tomato on *Datura stramonium* and concludes that incompatibility is in all probability not caused either by a defective union or by poisoning. The results suggests that wilting is caused by an unbalanced condition which develops gradually between the tomato graft and *Datura stramonium*.

Suzuki[164] found that the oxidation of phenols by partially purified enzyme and acetone powder occurred within D. tatula seedlings. Phenol oxidase activity was restricted mainly to the root and easily extracted. The phenol oxidase in the leaves seemed to be localized in the chloroplasts.

Sciuchetti and Iturrian[142] noticed the effects of dimethylsulfoxide (DMSO) and B 995 on the growth and metabolic products of *Datura innoxia*. They found that DMSO treated plants showed slight increase in concentration of alkaloid. In B995 treated plants the concentration of stem alkaloids increased by 56%.

Sciuchetti and Born[143] in their study on the effect of dimethylsulfoxide singly and in combination, with N-methylamino succinamic acid (B 995) or (2 chloroethyl) trimethylamonium chloride (ccc) on the growth and alkaloid biosynthesis of Datura tatual, noticed that DMSO caused reduction in plant weight and total alkaloid content per plant. The concentration of alkaloids in the roots was decreased. On the other hand B 995 and ccc induced significant reductions in plant height and total plant weight, but the concentration of alkaloids in the stem increased and in roots decreased. Phytotoxicity was seen in plants treated with CCC alone, or when used in combination with DMDSO.

Dallolio[30] investigated the effects of growth retarding compounds CCC and AMAB on the growth and alkaloid content of *D. stramonium*. He treated plants twice fortnightly with doses of 200 cc. to 2 m. solution of (2-choroethyl)-trimethyl amonium chloride (CCC)or (allyl). Trimethyle ammonium bromide (AMAB) and found that percentage concentration of total alkaloids in the leaves and roots of treated plants were similar with those of controls and therefore, he assumes that growth retarding chemicals do not interfere with the alkaloid synthesis.

Verzar-Petri records the formation of alkaloid spectrum in the different of *Datura* species at different stages of development.

The species have been bound to show same alkaloid spectrum, using quantitative analysis and paper chromatography. Differences occur in the time of appearance of the alkaloid components as well as in their relation to one another. He noticed, that alkaloid spectrum of Datura changes considerably during ontogenesis.

Parke and Pohloudek-Fabini[122] studied the chemistry and physiology of certain metabolically important acid especially the keto-acid metabolism of *D. stramonium* var. *stramonium*. They found that ketoglutaric and pyruvic acid contents were predominant over a 24 hour period.

Rowland and Gibson[134] observed the role of ascorbic acid oxidase in the hyoscyamine-scopolamine ratio in *Datura innoxia* and found that ascorbic acid oxidase activity was not involved in the alkaloid biosynthesis.

Maciejewska-Potapczykova and Jaworski[109] noticed the presence of phosphorous components and proteins in the secondary tumors of *D. stramonium*.

Sciuchetti and Neilsen[145] investigated the effects of B-hydroxyethylhydrazine on growth and alkaloid formation in *D. stramonium*. They found that spraying of aqueous solution of B hydroxyethylhydrazine (BOH) in strength of 1, 0-10, and 6.0001% brought about reduction of leaf-tops alkaloid to 45% but increased the root alkaloid by 61%. The total alkaloid content per plant was 26% of controls. In 0.0001% BOH sprayed groups increase of 11% in leaf tops, 103% in stems and 209% in roots were recorded.

Dallolia[29] noticed the influence of AMO-1618 on the growth and alkaloid content in *D. stramonium*. He noticed that plants sprayed with AMO-1618 became more compact, sturdier, leaves darker green and more thickened. AMO-1618 (4-hydroxy-5-isopropyl-2-methylphenyl-trimethyle ammonium chloride) treated plants showed no difference in the concentration of total alkaloids in roots and leaves than the controls.

Romoeike[133] in his investigations on the functions of shoot in the formation of alkaloids, found that several *Datura* species were able to demethylate hyoscyamine. This transformation could be connected with reactions appearing through metabolic degradation of norhyoscyamine. The demethylation of hyoscyamine in *Datura* seems to be differ than the demethylation of nicotine in *Nicotiana* species.

Cosson[27] observed the effect of light on alkaloid content during plant ontogenesis in *Datura*. He found that *D. tatula* and *D. metel* showed five ontogenic stages. He records that plants under intense daily 16-hour illumination revealed a sharp increase in scopolamine content during flowering.

El-hamidi et al[36] studied the effect of gamma radiations on *D. stramonium* var *inermis* grown in United Arab Republic and found that the increase of radiation doses. The plants which would could grow were comparatively weaker and shorter than the control. The number and weight of leaves and yield of fruits were less than the control at all stages of growth, flowering, fruiting of the treated plants occurred later than the control. In leaves and stems, alkaloid content increased with the irradiation of seeds. Maximum increase of 64 percent and 86 percent respectively was found in plants irradiated with 16.000 rad. over the control. Seeds and pericarps showed increase in alkaloid content even effected by small doses (12.000 rad.) of radiation.

Sciuchetti[146] noticed the effects of DMSO as a single factor and also in combination with various growth regulators. He found they effected the metabolic products within *Datura* species.

Kalichava[86] investigated the effects of electro-para-magnetic resonance on the free-radical states of tissues from *D. stramonium*.

Tetenyi[167] made some attempts to improve alkaloid contents within *D. stramonium* by using isotopic irradiation and found it could be raised to a certain level only.

Kraevoa[89] ascertained that grafting yielded plants which could produce seeds. He experimented on *Datura* plants and found grafting caused to significant changes in the hereditary variability of plants. His experiments indicate the fallacy of vegetative hybridization, that grafting could provide vegetative hybrids similar to those obtained from gametic union.

Momtezuma-de-Carvalho[118] was successful in inducing pollen tube formation with a single sperm nucleus by Nitrous oxide (N_2O). He observed that nitrous oxide effected the pollen tube mitosis.

Paun and Cucu[123] studied the harvest yields of *D. innoxia* obtained from medium lavigated chernozen. He could yield by delaying the harvest. Best quality drug was obtained from early harvest of stems and growing tips.

Verzar-Petri investigated the various morphological stages

of *D. metel* in Hungarian climatic conditions. He noticed that total alkaloid content in each organ, increased during different developmental stages. The development of originine, ornithine, protine glutamic acid etc. play an important part in the biogenesis of tropane alkaloids, while phenylalamine controls the ontogenetical rhythm of alkaloid contents.

Rohde and Brucker[131] noticed the effects of x-irradiation on growth and RNA nucleotide composition in *Datura* tissue cultures. They found X-irradiation (200 KV, 20mA 2 kR) effected increase of fresh weight of *D. innoxia* crown gall tumor (in vitro for 33 days). The irradiated tissues weighed 31 percent of untreated controls.

Cytidine phosphate content increased during growth, whereas the guanosine phosphate content decreased. They found that nucleotide composition ribosnal RNA changes during growth, the base composition of RNA from irradiated tissue was equal to that of controls.

Pharmacology

Bachrach et al[5] investigated the nature of protein responsible for the hemagglutinating activity of *D. metel* extract. They found that the active protein is a globulin similar to human globulin. They observed that active protein is not digested wither by trypsin or papain.

Bose et al[12] records the effect of Solanaceous lakaloids on the 5-hydroxy tryptamine content of rat brain.

Toxicity

Vorokhobov et al found 52 cases of thron-apple (*Datura*) poisoning.

Schumacher[147] noticed a case of poisoning of a child by intake of seeds of *Dautra Stramonium*. Toxicity resembling manical type of atropine intoxication.

Eichner et al[40] examined two case of belladonna poisoning. The belladonna came from tomatoes grown from *D. stramonium* graft.

Blood and Rudalph[11] records production of stimulants obtained from decoctions of *D. stramonium* to be toxic.

Brown[9] noticed that active constituents from *Datura stramonium* and *Atropa bellodonna* when used in combination causes hallucinogenic effect rather when belladonna is used singly.

Johnson[77] records the effect of Datura on his mental set up. He found it causes some mental aberrations.

Biosynthesis

Leete[92] studies the biosynthesis of tropic acid and pathway of alkaloids of *D. stramonium*. He fed two months old Datura plants with phenylamine labelled with C^{14} through roots. The yielded hyoscine and hyoscymine which upon hydrolysis gave tropic acid which contain all. This is suggestive of the fact that phenylalamine probably is a precursor in the synthesis of tropic acid by *Datura* plant.

Underhill records the biosynthesis of acid mostly of hyoscine and scopolamine in wild varieties of Datura.

Andrazekczuk and Kazkowski[2] in their investigations on biosynthesis of tropanealkaloids especially the esterification of tropine with tropic acid. They found that the root cultures of *D. metel* when fed with tropine and tropic acid showed significant increase of tropanalkaloids as compared to control roots. This fact signified that esterification of these two compounds takes place in plants producing tropane alkaloids. The unknown alkaloid was found in all samples of investigated roots. This base appeared in larger amounts in roots which were fed rather than the controls. In dynamic experiments it increases, the largest during first three days of investigation. This fact according to them can be a precursor of hyscyamine and is produced directly from tropine. The data obtained suggest the possibility of the reaction of epoxydation of hyoscyamine to scopolamine in the roots of *D. metel*.

Turner studies the biosynthesis of scopolamine in *D. stramonium*.

Evans and Griffin[44] in their investigations on metabolic pathways in *D. innoxia* found that the plants incorporate C^{14} O_2 more rapidly into tygloyl groups of the ditigloyl ester alkaloids than into the hydroxy tropane moiety of the molecule 3, 6-Ditigloyloxytropane fed to the leaves of *D. innoxia* and *D. cornigera*, undergoes a stepwise hydrolysis by which 3-hydroxy-6-

tigloyloxytropane is found in both the species. In addition 3, 6-dithydroxytropane is produced in *D. innoxia* while 6-hydroxy-3-tigloyloxytropane in *D. cornigera*. 7-hydroxy-3, 6-diti-glyoloxy-tropane undergoes a similar hydrolysis in the aerial organs of *Datura* and gives rise to meteloidine; in *D. innoxia* and *D. ferox*. Another monoester and teloidene have been derived from it, In D. innoxia 3,6, 7-triditigloyloxytropane being an intermediate in its breakdown. This, in conjunction with other evidence suggests that meteloidine and 3-hydroxy-6-tigloly-oxytropane are formed in the leaves of normal plants.

Leete[93] records in his findings on biosynthesis of hyoscyamine, in *D. stramonium* that orthinine-2-C^{14} yield tropine labelled at C-1.

Kaczkowski[82,83] studied the enzymic synthesis and hydrolysis of hyscyamine in-vitro of some datura species.

Gibson and danquiest[57] in their studies on biosynthetc pathways of alkaloids noticed that *Datura innoxia* root cultures absorb di-hydroxyprotine-2C^{14} and distribute it to hyoscymine and scopolamine as well as to other alkaloids. The low level of incorporation suggest an indirect route and not a direct incorporation from an exogenous amino acid pool.

Liebisch et al[96, 97] found that the biosynthesis of tropane alakaloids in the species of *Datura* brings about sterospectifically incorporated ornithin-(2-C^{14}) be considered as a physiologically possible precursor of the tropane alkaloids.

Neu-mann and Schroter[120] records N-emthylornithin to be a preliminary step of the pyrollidine ring in tropane alkaloids obtained in *D. stramonium* and *D. metel*.

Madan et al[107] suggests the location of alkaloids in the capsules and seed portions of *Datura* species.

Ghosal[52] carried out biogenesis of tropic acid obtained from *D. stramonium* using carbon-monoxide insertion reaction. Evans and Wooley[45] studied the biosynthesis of tiglolesters in *D. meteloids*.

Burdykina-Shekhter[15] in his investigations on the mechanism of origin of alkaloids in *Datura innoxia* found that D. innoxia grafted on tomato plants do not contain alkaloids, while tomato plants grafted on *D. innoxia* root does contain scopolamine and hyoscyamine. The root consequently plays a leading role in the formation of alkaloids in *D. innoxia*.

Jindra et al[73, 74] observed the role f enzymatic activity in alkaloid synthesis of D. stromanium and *Papaver sominiferum*. THey noticed in *P. sominiferum* tryosine hydroxylation, phenylalamine trioxine, 3,4-deoxyphenylalamine and glutaminic acid decarboxylation. Secondary oxidative reactions which are calalysed by phenol oxidases are all enzymatic reactions. Investigation of transminase activity only in the resette stage up to flowering time. These findings throw additional light on the sequence timing and identification of intermediary reactions.

Leete and Murrill[94] experimented to observe biosynthesis of tiglic acid moiety of meteloidene in *D. metaloids*.

Verzar-Ptri investigated the formation of amino acid spectrum during the ontogenesis in the some *Datura* species. He observed that there is a general inverse correlation between the ornithine-proline-arginine cycle and total alkaloid content.

Woolley records some observations on the biosynthesis of the tigloyl esters of *Datura*.

Neumann and Schroter[119, 120] found N-methyl-ornithin as preliminary step of pyrollidine rings in pyridine and tropane alkaloids while investigating alkaloids obtained from *D. stramonium* and *D. metel*. Jindra et al [74, 75] investigated transimnation reaction in the biosynthesis of *Datura*. Opium, Nicotiana and Lobelia alkaloids. They found that enzymatically catalysed transmination reactions enabled the transformation of aminoacids to the corresponding oxo compounds and some of the results lead to be better understanding of mechanism of biochemical processes involved directly in alkaloid biosynthesis.

Liebisch et al[97,98] studied the biosynthesis of the tropane-alkaloids. They found that the labelled proline. Glutamic acid, N-acetyl glutamic acid and pyrrolid-2-one-5-carbo-oxylic acids are less efficient precursors of the pyrollidine moety of tropane alkaloids in *D. metel* and *D. stramonium* than pubriscine and ornithine. Proline (5-C)^{14} seems to be sterospecifically incorporated. Experiments with C^{14} N^{15} double labelled ornithine, show that the heterocyclic nitrogen of tropane nucleus and proline is derived mainly from the-amino group, N^{15} content of glutamic acid (2-C^{14}) N^{15}) is lost during incorporation.

Schutte and Liebisch[138] added to the knowledge of the biosynthesis of tropane alkallids. They point out formation of tropic acid from phenylalamine-1-C^{14}, 2-H^3.

Gibson, C.A. and Youngken[58] carried out biosynthesis of tropic acid in *Datura innoxia*. They fed the plants with Phenylalamine-UL^{14}=C, Phenylalamine-1, 3=^{14}C and Shiumic acid-UL-^{14} C and extracted radio active hyoscyamine and scopolamine. These were degraded to determine the position of radio active carbon of the tropic acidmoiety. The results indicated that all the carbon of tropic acid are derived from carbons of phenylalamine and carboxyl carbon of tropic acid is derived from the carboxyl carbon of phenylalamine by way of some intramolecular shift mechanism.

Jindra[75] recounts the investigations done on biosynthesis pathway of alkaloids in *Datura stramonium* and *Papaver somniferum*. He records the use of precursors of enzyme activity analyses to elucidate tropane and opium alakloid biosynthesis.

Leete and Nelson[95] studied the Biosynthesis of the telodine moiety of meteloidene in *Datura meteloides* and found that DL-ornithine-2^{14} C when administered in three months old *D. meteloides* plants, the meteloidine isolated 12 days later was radioactive (0.3 percent incorporation). On systematic degradation carried out on the alkaloid they found that all the activity was located at one or both of the bridge head carbons (C-1 and C-5) of teloidene moiety of alkaloid. These results are in consistent with the hypothesis that teloidene is formed by the hydroxylation of tropine perhaps iva 6, 7 dehydrotrophine.

Phytochemistry

Ellert[38] extracted scopolamine from *D. metel.* he found it contained on an average 0.12% alkaloids including 0.090% scopolamine. He was able to obtain 3.51 gm. of crystalline scopolamine hydrobromide from 4550 gm of pulverized and dried leaves.

Pawelczak[124] found that percentage of tropine alkaloids varied with the vegetative stages of the plant. She noticed that it was greatest in leaves before plant blossoms. In subsequent phases of vegetative growth a gradual decreased of alkaloid content occurs.

Lukasiak[104] investigated the amount and types of carbohydrates produced within stems tissues of *D. stramonium*. He found 5 groups of carbohydrates namely mono, di an triscсharides, dextrines mucliages and parts of pectic substances. Carbohydrates of the first, third and fourth groups decreased while the remaining types increased in the tumours caused by *Agro-bacterium*.

Alkaloids

Demaggio et al[31, 32] devised a new method of isolation of alkallids by using ultrasonic energy, where-in two to four hours of conventional maceration of the tissues was followed by two hours of ultrasonic extraction with a 20 KC/S generator gave a significant increase in the total alkaloid recovery as compared with controls. The evidence suggest that during maceration ultrasound liberatese alkaloids from bound sites thus hastening their rates of diffusion into the solvent and during extraction it accelerates the physical separation of alkaloids from the grounded plant material.

Olaechea and Arraras[121] suggests that *D. ferox* leaves could be substituted from *Atrops belladonna* and *D. stramonium*. They point out that *d. ferox* leaves can be good source of raw materials for obtaining scopolamine.

Chan-Wen-Nuei and Stabe[20] records chemical similarities within the *Datura* tissue cultures using thin layer chromatography.

Sileva[166] studied the protein composition of the seeds of various species of *Datura* and formulated a phylogenetic system based on the solubility of these proteins in various solvents.

Shah and Khanna[249, 150] records the presence of hyoscyamine, hyoscine and meteloidine in the leaves and roots of D. innoxia while they record presence of hyoscyamine and hyoscine in flowers pericarps and seeds. They found roots to contain 7-hydroxy-3, 6-ditigloyloxytropane (-)-3 68-diliglylo tropane, tropine and pseudotropine.

Evans at al[46] noted finding of scopolamine as the principal alkaloid together with smaller quantities of hyoscyamine, Nor-scopolamine, Aposcopolamine and other uncharacterized basis in the aerial parts of *D. sanquinea*. They were able to obtain 3, 69, ditigloyloxytropane, 3,6-ditigloyloxytropane, 3, 6-ditigloloxy-tropane-7-ol, hyoscine hyoscyamine (and or atropine) and smaller amounts of other alkaloids from the roots.

Wallis studied the alkallids of *D. sanquinea* and records finding in the seeds of Peruvian plant present of hyoscine.

Verzar-Petre investigated the composition of alkaloid spectra in *Datura* varieties during ontogenesis. He records the presence of cuskhigirine, hyoscyamine, scopalamine, 7-hydroxy-tropane, metaloidene and two other unknown alkaloids.

Shaha and Saoji[151-153] estimated the alkaloidal contents from the aerial parts of *D. arborea*. They record presence of hyoscine and hyoscyamine in leaves, flowers and stems. All parts contain higher percentage of hyoscine than hyosyamine in the ratio of 2:1. They found one unidentified alkaloid in chloroform fraction.

Further they record isolation of (–) 3, 6-Ditigloyloxaytropane, 7 hydroxy, 3, 6-ditiglyloxytropane, tropine, hyoscine and hyoscyamine from *D. arborea* roots. Ammoniacial chloroform elyate along with topane shows presence of pseudotropine.

Griffin[62] records presence of scopolamine and metaloidine forom leaves of peach flowered form of Datura (*D. candida*) together with small quantities of nor scopolamine nor hyoscyamine and an unidentified base. Hyoscyamine was not detected in the leaves, on the other hand flowers contained scopolamine, nor scopolamine, and meteloidine. Scopolamine was the principal alkaloid. Stems showed scopolamine, hyoscyamine and meteloidine. From roots (–) 3,6-ditigloyloxytropane, 3, 6-ditiglyoloxytropane 7-ol, scopolamine hyoscyamine atropine, nor-hyoscyamine meteloidine, tropine and unidentified bases, were isolated.

In young roots, ditigloylesters were present of these, (–) 3,6-diligloyl-oxy-tropane occurred in large amounts, while 3,6-ditigloloxytropane 7.01 was a minor component, of the alkaloids.

Yamada et al noticed the non-enzymic transformation of phenylalamine to tropic acid. They could obtain acid moety of ester alkaloids from *D. stramonium*.

References

1. Akisue, Gokithi : Rev. Fac. Farm. Bigin. U.N. Sao. Paulo. 2 (2), 147, (1965).
2. Andrazejczuk, J and J. Kaczkowski : Acta Soc. bot. Polon. 31(3), 461, (1962).
3. Ambrose, D.G., and L.A. Sciuchetti : Jour. Pharmaceut. Sci. 51(10), 934, (1962).
4. Avery, A.G., S. Satina and J. Reitsema : *Balakeslee* the *genus Datura*, New York. (1959).
5. Bachrach, U.D. Be rechyahy and J. Gurevitch : Jour Immunolog 82(2), 116 (1959).

6. Bailey D.R. : Queensland. Agr. Jour. 94(4), 233 (1964).
7. Barclay A.A. : Bot. Mus. Leaflet. Hav. Univ. 18(6), 245, (1959).
8. Bennet, J.H., and L.A. Sciuchetti : J. Pharm. Sci. 53(10), 1254, (1964).
9. Brown T : J. Amer. Med. Assoc. 203(8), 606, (1968).
10. Blattney, C.J. Brcak, J. Pozdena, J. Dlabola, J. Limberk, and V.B. Jnansky : Phyto. Path. Zeit. 22(4), 381, (1954).
11. Blood, F.R. and G. R. Rudolph : Nat. Acad. Sci. Nat. Res. Counc. Publ. 1354, 62, (1967).
12. Bose, B.C., M.A. Matin, R. Viyavergiya and L. Lahiri : J. Pharm. Pharmacol. 18(10), 690 (1966).
13. Bristol. M.L. : Harv. Univ. Bot. Mus. Leafl.21(8), 229, (1966).
14. Borges, Maria de lourdes : Agron. Lusitana 25(2), 63, (1963).
15. Burdykina-Shekhter, E.A. : Rest. Resursy. 2(1) 56, (1966).
16. Brucker, W. and W.A.K. Schmidit: Ber. Deutsch. Bot. Ges. 72(8), 321 (1959).
17. Gaesar W : Pharma. 13(3) : 167, (1958).
18. Carroll, T.W. and T.A.A Shalla : Phytopath, 55(8), 928, (1965).
19. Carroll, T.W : Phytopath, 56(12), 1348, (1966).
20. Chan, wen-Nuei and E.J. Staba : Amer. Pharm. Assoc. 27, 67(1964).
21. Chan, Wen-Nuei and E.J. Staba : Lloydia 28(1), 55, (1965).
22. Chiu, Ren-Jong and W.H. Sill. : Phytopath 53(1), 69, (1963).
23. Chiu, Ren-Jong and W.H. Sill : Plant. Dist. Report 43(7), 690, (1959).
24. Chiu, R.J. and W.H. Sill. : Phytopath. 50(9), 632, (1960).
25. Caldwell, E.L. and L.A. Sciuchetti : J. Pharmaceut. Sci. 52(11), 1062, (1963).
26. Cohen, S. and F.E. Nitzany : Phytopath. 56 (10), 1127, (1966).
27. Cosson, L : Herba Hung. 5(2/3), 157, (1966).
28. Dachyshyn, O.T. Farm. Zh. 20(4), 41, (1965).
29. Dallolio, G : G. Bot. Ital. 71(1/2), 23, (1964).
30. Dallolio, G: G. Bot. Ital. 72(2/3), 334, (1965).
31. Demaggio, A.E., J.A. Lott. and R.J. Gerraughty : Nature 199(4900), 1292, (1963).
32. Demaggio, A.E. and J.A. Lott : J. Pharm. Sci. 53(8), 945, (1964).
33. Dewolf, G.P.: Baileya 4(1), 12, (1956).
34. Denert, S. : Feddes. Rep. Spec. Nov. Reg. Veg. 57(3), 231, (1955).
35. Dimitri-Jevic, B : Zast. Bilja 17(91-92), 315, (1966).
36. El-hamidi, A.M. Saleh and H. Hamidi : Abhanol. Deut Akad. Wiss. Berlin, (1966 (3), 567, (1966).
37. El-hamidi, A.M. Saleh and H. Hamidi : Abhanol. Deut. Akad. Wiss. Berlin. (1966 (3), 567, (1966).
38. Ellert, H : Diss. Pharmaceut. 7, 129, (1956).
39. Elze, H. and E. Teuscher : Flora. Allg. Bot. Zig. Abt. a Physiol. Biochem. (Jena), 158(1), 127, (1967).
40. Eichner, E.R., J.M. Gunsolus and J.F. Powers : J. Amer. Med. Asso. 102 (9), 695, (1967).
41. Eshel, Y : Weeds, 15(2), 147, (1967).
42. Evans, W.C. and W.J. Griffin : Lloydia 25(3), 139, (1962).
43. Evans, W.C. and W.J. Griffin : J Pharm. and Pharmacol. 16(5), 337 (1964).
44. Evans, W.C. and W.J. Griffin : Phytochemistry 3(4), 503 (1964).
45. Evans, W.C. and J.G. Woolley : Jour. Pharm. Pharmacol. 17, 375, (1965).
46. Evans, W.C. Valeria, A.M. M. Pe Than : Planta Med. 13(3), 353, (1965).
47. Erasmus, S.P. : Mededl. Landbouwhogesch. Wageningen. 65(2), 43, (1965).

48. Eskarous, J.K. : Advan. Frontiers Plant Sci. 19, 157, (1968).
49. Fites, R.C., F.W. Slife and J.B. Hansons: Weeds, 12(3), 180, (1964).
50. Force, D.: Ann. Entomol. Soc. Amer. 59(6), 1112, (1966).
51. Fosberg, F.R. : Taxon 8(2), 52, (1959).
52. Ghosal, S : Sci and Cult. 31(7), 370, (1965).
53. Gerasimenko, I.I. : Bot. Zhur. 47(2), 282, (1962).
54. Gerasimenko, I.I. : Rast. Resur. 3(1), 74, (1967).
55. Gibson. M.R. and E.A. Abbott : Lloydia, 26(3), 125, (1963).
56. Gibson, M.R. and D.I. French : Lloydia, 27(1), 47 (1964).
57. Gibson, M.R. and G.A. Danquist : J. Pharm. Sci. 54(10), 1526, (1965).
58. Gibson, G.A. and H.W. Youngken : J. Pharm. Sci. 56(7), 854, (1967).
59. Guha, S. and S.C. Maheshwari : Nature 212 (5057), 97, (1966).
60. Guha, S. and S.C. Maheshwari : Nature, 204 (4957), , 497, (1964).
61. Gugliada, M.E., A. Soriano and S. Burkart. Can. J. Bot 45(3), 377, (1967).
62. Griffin, W.J.: Planta Medica 14(4) : 468, (1966).
63. Gross, D. and H.R. Schutte: Arch, Pharm. u Ber. Der. Deutsch. Phramazent, Gassel. 296(1), 6, (1963).
64. Hayashi, T. and Chiakimatsu : Virology 33(1), 47, (1967).
65. Hildebrand, D.C., J.P. Thompson and M.N. Schroth : Phytopath. 56(3), 365, (1966).
66. Hirst, J.M. and W.C. Moore : Plant Pathol. 6(2), 76, (1957).
67. Horvath, J. : Acta Phytopathol. Acad. Sci. Hung : 1(3/4), 333, (1966).
68. Horvath, J. Acta PHytopathol. 1(1/2), 125, (1966).
69. Ismailov, N.M. : Gast. Resur. 3(1), 53, (1967).
70. Jain, R.K. Curr. Sci. 27(10), 394, (1958).
71. James, R.P. and L.A. Sciuchetti : J. Pharm. Sci. 53(9), 1093, (1964).
72. Jankulov, J : C.R. Acad. Bulg. Sci. 20(3), 225, (1967).
73. Jindra, A., P. Kovacs, Z. Pittner O. M. Svova and H.S. Mogrovicova : Herba Hung. 5(2/3), 30, (1966).
74. Jindra, A., P. Kovacs, H. Smogrovica and M. Svova : Lloydia 30(2), 158, (1967).
75. Jindra, A ; Acta Fac. Pharm. Bochemo, Slov. 13, 7, (1967).
76. Jidnra, A. and E. John Staba : Phytochemistry 7(1), 79, (1968).
77. Johnson, C: Int. J. Neuropschiat. 3(3), 268, (1967).
78. Kahn, P. and R. Bartels : Phytopathol. 58(5), 587, (1968).
79. Karnick, C.R. and M.D. Saxena : Proc. 55th Ind. Sci. Cong. Abst. 407, (1968).
80. Kardos, J : Acta. Biol. Acad. Sci. Hung. 14(4), 285, (1964).
81. Karkoszka, A.H. Krasowska and K. Rogoyska : Diss. Pharamaceut., 9(4), 287, (1957).
82. Kaczkowski, J : Bull, Acad. Bol. Sci, Ser. Sci. Biol. 12(9), 375, (1964).
83. Kaczkowski, J : Abhandl, Deut. Akad. Wiss. Berlin. 1966(3), 521, (1965).
84. Kaul, B.L. Cytologia. 33(1), 17, (1968).
85. Kalichava, G.S. Loginoya, L.N. and L.N. Saldan : Soobshch, akad, Nauk, Gruz, SSR. 41(2), 431, (1966).
86. Kalichava, G.S. : Soobshch Akad. Mauk. Gruz, SSR. 42(3), 693, (1966).
87. Kalichava, G.S. and L.N. Loginova : Soobshch Akad. Nauk, Gruz, SSR. 41(3), 693, (1966).
88. Klesser, P. : Bothalia 9(1), 173, (1966).
89. Kraevoa, S. Ya : Izv. Akad. Nauk, SSR. SER, Biol. 1, 63, (1967).
90. Kolodziejski, J. and A. Kuleszyna : Acta. Polon. Pharm. 16, 287, (1959).

91. Krogerus, V : Arch. Soc. Zool. Bot Fenn. Venamo : 17(1), 19, (1962).
92. Leete, E. : Jour. Amer. Chem. Soc. 82(3), 612, (1960).
93. Leete, E. Tetrahedron. Lett. 23/24, 1619, (1964).
94. Leete, E. and J.B. Murrill : Tetrahedron Lett. 18, 1727, (1967).
95. Leete, E. and S.J. Nelson : Phytochem, 8, 413, (1969).
96. Liebisch, H.W., H. ramin, I Schoffinius and H.R. Schutte : Z. Naturforsch. 20(12), 1183, (1965).
97. Liebisch, H.W. : Abhanol Deut. Akad. Wiss. Berlin. 3,525, (1965).
98. Liebisch, H.W. and Horst R. Schutte : Z. Planzen. Physiol. 57(2), 435, (1967).
99. Little, T.M. Bot. Rev. 24(5), 318 (1958).
100. Linsley, E.G: Jour New York, Entmol. Soc. 68(1), 13, (1960).
101. Lovrekovich, L. and G. Loebenstein : Phytopath, 56(5), 578, (1966).
102. Loebenstein, G. and A. Frankross : Virology 20(3), 507, (1963).
103. Loebenstein, G., Schlomit. R. and Tirzah Vam. Praagh : Proc. Internat. Conf. Plant Virus. Wagenigen. 5, (1965).
104. Lukasiak, H : Acta Soc. Bot. Polon. 30(2), 263, (1961).
105. Lukasiak, H. Acta. Soc. Bot. Polon. 32(3), 505, (1963).
106. Lynn. M.J : Irish, Nat. Jour. 13(5), 107, (1960).
107. madan, C.L., U.S. Gupta, V.S. Prabhakar and B.M. Kapoor : Naturwissenschaften 53(4), 109, (1966).
108. Madan, C.L. U.S. Gupta and R.K. Khanna Curr. Sci. 35(12), 311, (1966).
109. Maciejewska-Potapczykova, W.A. Jaworski : Acta Soc. Bot. Pol. 34(2), 153, (1965).
110. Maniquis, E.P. : Diss. Absts. 20(8), 3331, (1960).
111. Manigault, P. and G. beaud : Rev. Roumaine. Biol. Ser. Bot. 11(1/3), 135, (1966).
112. Manigault, P. and G. Beaud : Inst. Pasteur. (Paris). Amn. 112(4), 445, (1967).
113. Massiaen, C.M. and J. Marrow : Ann. Epiphyt. (Paris). 18. h.s., 173, (1967).
114. Massini, P; Acta Bot. Neerlandica 6(4), 434, (1957).
115. Miyomoto, S.Y. Miyamoto : Sci. Rep. Hy. Ogo. Univ. Agr. Ser. Plant Prot. 7(2), 51, (1966).
116. Morgan, O.D. : plant Disease Rep. 42(2), 222, (1958).
117. Mothes, K., A. Romeike and H.B. Schrother : Naturawiss, 42(8), 214, (1955).
118. Montezuma-de-CArvalho : Euphtica 16(2), 190, (1967).
119. Numann, D. and H.B. Schroter : Abhandl, Akad, Wiss, Berlin, 3, 161, (1966).
120. Neumann, D. and H.B. Schroter : Tetrahedron. left. 30, 3541, (1966).
121. Olacchea, V.P. and E.G. Arraras : Rev. Fac. Cienc. Quim. Univ. Nac. la. Plata 33, 37 (1961).
122. Parke, E.R. Pohloudek-Fabini : Pharmazie, 19(9), 610, (1964).
123. Paun, E.V. Cucu : Probl. Agr. 11, 29, (1966).
124. Pawelczak, I. Diss. Pharmaceut. 7, 187, (1956).
125. Perez, A.F. : colloq. Unternationause, Centre, Nat. Reché, Sci. 144, 89, (1966).
126. Pozeulo, J.M. and M. Rozario de Felie : Farmacognosis (Madrid.) 25 (1/2), 51, (1965).
127. Puiseziu-Dao, S.D. Gibelo and D. Hoursiandouneubrun : Cr. He. Bd. Seances, Acad. Sci. Ser. d. Sci. Natur. (Paris). 265(5), 406, (1967).
128. pratsap Singh and B. L. Kaul : INd. J. Exp. Bio. 5(5), 128, (1967).
129. Quantz, L : Phytopathol. Zetischer. 23(2), 209, (1955).
130. Reifman, V.G. : Bot Zhur. 47(4), 577, (1962).
131. Rohde, H.G. and W. Brucker : Z. Pflanzen. Physiol. 58(4), 327, (1968).

132. Romeike A : Kultur pflanze 10, 140, (1962).
133. Romeike A : ;Flora Allg. Bot. Zeitung. (Jena). 154(1).
134. Rowland, H.L. and M.R. Gibson : J. Pharm. Sci. 55, 1354. (1966).
135. Sandberg F : Colloq. Internat. Centre, Nat. Reche, Sci. 144, 49, (1966).
136. Sanchez, R.A., A. Soriano. and Slabnik : can. J. Bot. 45(3), 371, (1967).
137. Schuster-G : Wiss. Z. Karl. Marx. Univ. Leipzig. Math. natur. Reihe. 15(1), 101, (1966).
138. Schutte, H.R. and H. Liebisch : Z Pflanzen. Physiol. 57(5), 440, (1967).
139. Sciuchetti L.A : Pharmaceut. Sci. 53(1), 61-62 (1964).
140. Sciuchetti L.A. A. Hisatomy and A.N. Masound : J. Pharm. Sci. 54(3), 403, (1965).
141. Sciuchetti, L.A. and N.C. Mingis : Iloydia 28(3), 230, (1965).
142. Sciuchetti, L.A. and R.C. Iturrian : J. Pharm. Sci. 54(10), 1477, (1965).
143. Sciuchetti, L.A. and A.E. Born : J. Pharm. Sci. 54(2). 285, (1965).
144. Sciuchetti, L.A. and G.G. Hutchinson : Lloydia 29(4), 368, (1966).
145. Sciuchetti, L.A. and G.K. Nielsen : J. Pharm. Sci. 56(2) 244, (1967).
146. Sciuchetti, L.A. : Ann. N.Y. Acad. Sci. 141(1), 139, (1967).
147. Schumacher, M : Med. J. Aust. 521 (15), 547, (1965).
148. Shah, C.S. and P.N. Khanna : Ind. J. Pharm. 27(8), 222. (1965).
149. Shah, C.S. and P.N. Khanna : Lloydia 28(1), 71, (1965).
150. Shah, C.S. and P.N. Khanna : J. Pharm. Pharmacol. 17(2), 115, (1965).
151. Shah, C.S. and .AN. Saoji : Ind. J. Pharm. 29(7), 199, (1966).
152. Shah, C.S. and A.N. Saoji : Planta Med. 14(4), 465, (1966).
153. Shah, C.S. and A.N. Saoji : Ind. J. Pharm. 29(3), 95, (1967).
154. Sharma P.C. : Nat. Acad. Sci. Ind Proc. Sec. B. Bio. Sci. 34(4), 476, (1965).
155. Shorin, V.A., O.K. Rossolimo and E.S. Kudrina : Antibiotik 1(1), 15, (1956).
156. Skogen A : Blyttia 22 (2), 78 (1964).
157. Shpilenya, S.E. : Doklady, Akad. Nauk. SSSR, 141 (3), 751, (1962).
158. Sinha A.S. and K.C. Verma : Ind. J. Pharm. 28(1), 3, (1966).
159. singh D.V. and R.S. Mathus : Sci. and Cult. 30(12), 604, (1964).
160. Singh, D.N. and R. Fatima : genet. Iber. 18(3-4), 270, (1966).
161. Sullivan G. and M.R. Gibson : J. Pharm. Sci. 53 (9), 1058, (1964).
162. Summanwar, A. Diss. Abstr. 25 (12), 6873, (1965).
163. Summanwar, A.S. and W.J. Hooker : Phytopathol 54(8), 909, (1964).
164. Suzuki, Y :.Phyton, Rev. Int. Bot. Exp. 21(1), 7 : (1964).
165. Soriano, A. R.A. Sanxhe and B.A. de Eiberg : Can. J. Bot. 42(9), 1189, (1964).
166. Sileva, M.N. : Ref. Zh. Biol. 4, 138, (1964).
167. Staba, E.J. and A. Jindra : J. Pharm. Sci. 57(4), 701, (1968).

VII

Plants Used in Ayurvedic System of Medicine for Madhumeya (Diabetes)

Disease, decay and death have co-existed with life. The method of study of different diseases developed simultaneously in several parts of the world. Different systems of medicine came to be recognised with different civilisations. (Pyke,[8] Collier[4] and Drash[6]). India developed its own unique type of system which stood the test of several centuries and is in practice even today in most of the Indian villages.

Ayurveda, has a vast medical literature with many classics to its credit. Charaka Samhita[2], Sushtruta Samhita[9, 10]. Asthanga Hridaya[1] and others are used as quide lines by Ayurvedic physicians.

This paper deals with the "Muthra roga" ailment, termed as "Madhumeha" or Diabetes.

Madhumeha : (Diabetes) : What it is?

In modern terminology, it is recognised as an acute disorder presenting copious micturation, wasting and thirst, progressing eventually to coma and death (Jarret[7]). It is a disease due to insulin deficiency (Taylor[13], Collier[4]).

Ayurvedic Concepts

Sushruta[9], mansions that most of the urino-genital diseases ("Muthra-roga") have their origin in the disturbances of "Vayu" (gases) within the bowels.

The concept is that "Jatha rogni" is mainly responsible for proper digstion of food (Shastri[11]). This "Jatha rogni" is a gasses exchange which controls the internal temperatures of organs and is connected with digestion. It is further pointed out that human body has nine internal gas orifices for this gaseous exchange (Vayu) Shastri[11]).

The sounds produced by the heart pulsation have been interpreted differently in Caraka which states that "Jwala Sabda" is the cause in keeping the pulsating movements of heart. "Vayus" have been classified into several groups as per their actions within different parts of body.

Caraka[2] further mentions that "Samana Agni" is channelled out into the skin, any disturbance within it brings out "Bhrajaka pitta" or skin diseases (Shastri[11]). Furthermore, it is pointed out that any disturbance in the bowels is clearly indicated in the eye ball. This is due to connections of `Vayu channels' to the eye. In `Madhumeha' (Diabetes), vision is generally disturbed (Shastri[11]).

Food is first digested by "Jatharagni". Then five "Bhuta-agni" react bringing out selective absorption, viz. `Parthiv agni' brings about digestion of fatty oils and carbohydrates; "Jaliya-agni" acts on milk, fruits and other fluids while the remaining food is acted upon by "Taijas Agni. Any disturbances of "Taijas Agni", leads to unbalance of "Vatta", "Pitha" and Kapha, which in turn, results in flow of sugar in the blood stream and thrown out in urine i.e. "Madhumeya".

Healing Technique

Ayurvedic physicians use combination of fresh crude plant drug extracts with control on the type of food taken during treatment. This has resulted in bringing about the stoppage to sugar from the body. It would be interest to note that active principles within fresh plant extracts differ much in potency and activity, than when active principles are produced by hot chemical solvents. Their biochemical activity completely changes.

A few Indian drug plants used in indigenous system of medicine as a remedy for "Madhumeya" are enumerated below :

1. Meshashring : *Gymnema sylvestre* R. Br. (Asclepiadaceae). *Chemistry* : Leaves, if chewed, have the property to deaden the taste of sweetness. This is due to presence of gynemin, the potassinm salt of gymnemic acid. Leaf also contains 7% resin. hentriacontane, pentatria contane, tartaric acid and anthraquinones have been isolated (Indian Med. Res. Mem. 16, 1930).

Pharmacology : Extracts of leaf stimulate the cardiovascular system, increase secretion of urine, stimulates the uterus and produce hypoglycaemia. The hypoglycaemic effects set in soon the administration of the drug, whether by mouth or by injection, lasts for a variable time and is not necessarily proportionate to the dose, it is never excessive. The drug has no direct action on carbohydrate metabolism, but acts indirectly through stimulation of insulin secretion of the pancreas. The purgative action of the leaf is accounted for by its contents of anthraquinones. The drug appears to be useful in checking glycosuria when administered in doses of 2 to 4 gm of dry leaf. The leaf ash is high (11.45%) (Indian Med. Res. Mem. 16, 1930; J. Sci. Industr. Res. 16A, 1957).

Distribution : Konkan, Deccan, West Ghats

2. "Sushavi: (*Momordica charantia* Linn) (Cucurbitaceae).

Juice of leaves, emetic, purgative, given in bilious affections also.

Chemistry : Fruits contain highly aromatic essential oil, carotene glycosides, saponin, and alkaloid momoridicine (Amer. J. Pharm. 261, 1941).

Pharmacology : The drug from fruits exhibited hypoglycaemic action when tested on rabbits. The effect being more marked with a crude crystalline substance extracted from the drug (Rivera, 1941). It is used as an antidiabetic in Puerto Rica (J. Publ. Heth, 19, 196, 1943).

Distribution : Cultivated throughout India.

3. Astmabayda (*Aerva lanats* Juss), (Amaranthaceae)

The whole herb is used in medicine. It is considered "Sita yam". It is used in "Rakta pittam" (haematemesis) and diabetes.

Pharmacology : It is diuretic ("Mutrala").

Distribution : Throughout India.

4. "Satavari" (*Asparagus racemosus* Willd), (Libaceae). *Chemistry* : Root contains-sitosterol and 2 more crystalline compounds, Saraspogenin and a new sapogenin B isolated.

Pharmacology : Some pronounced galactotropic activity, blocking of uterine activity, both spontaneous and induced by acetylcholine and oxytoxin.

Ayurveda : Preparation known as "Satavari guda" is used in didabetes jaundice and other urinary disorders.
Distribution : Throughout India, in Himalayas upto 1000 m.

5. "Guduchi" (Tinospora cordifolia Willd), Miers (Menispermaceae).
Chemistry : Berberine, a bitter substance (Bull. Inst. bot. Buitenz. XIV, II, 1902; Indian J. Med. Res. 663, 1932). Stem contains 0.1% bitter substance, another bitter principle and a neutral substance (J. Univ. Bombay, 89, 1941): fresh stems gave crude giloin and giloinin (J. Sci. Indust. Res. 11, 58, 1949).

Bhava Misra quotes that Guduchi overcomes three Dosa, Ama and Jaundice.
Distribution : Throughout India.

6. "Amalaki" (*Phyuanthus emblica* Linn), syn : Emblica officinalis Gaertin (Euphorbiaceae).
Chemistry : Fruit rich in vitamin C (Biochem. J. 1014 (1936). Seeds contain fixed oil, phosphatides and essential oil (J. Sci. industr. Res. 888, 1951). Fruits, bark, leaves rich in tannin (Indian For. heaft. No. 72, 9, 1944). Leaves contain phyllanthin, Vitamin C. Fresh roots used as remedy for jaundice.
Ayurveda : Amalaki juice with turmeric powder and honey cures. *Diabetes insipedus*.
Distribution : Common in mixed deciduous forests of India.

7. "Nira-brahmi" : *Bacopa monnieri* (Linn.) Pennell (Scrophulariaceae).
Chemistry : Leaves alkaloid brahmine, three bases isolated, B_1 oxalate, B_2, oxalate, B_3 chloroplatinate and a sterol (Indian J. Pharm. 91, 1944): contains alkaloid herpestine (Quart. J. Pharm. 137, 1947).

There is another plant which goes by the same name : *Centella asiatica* (Linn) Urban syn. Hydrocotyle asiatica Linn (Umbelliferae).
Chemistry : Leaves contain bitter substance (J. Pharm, Anvers 47, 1855) ; fresh leaves a glucoside asiaticoside 0.07 to0.12% (Bull. Sci. Pharm, 186, 1941), essential oil, fatty oil, sitosterol, tannin and resinous substance isolated from herb (Proc. Indian Acad. Sci. 54, 1937); alkaloid hydrocotylin (Quart. J. Pharm. 135, 1947).

Pharmacology : Asiaticoside active in Leprosy; asiaticoside and oxy-asiaticoside used in tuberculosis (Nature, London 601, 1945), insecticidal (Chem. Abstr. 2202, 1947), a bitter principle, vellarine, pectic acid and resin present in leaves and roots (ascorbic acid present Chem. Abstr. 2223, 1941).
Ayurveda : The drug cures dermatosis, anaemia, diabetes and insanity.
Distribution : In hills at wet places, near ponds.

8. Suvarnaka (Aragavadhah), *Cassia fistula* Linn (Leguminosae).
Chemistry : Leaves contain anthraquinone derivatives and very little tannan (Bol. Acad. Farm. Rio. de.J. 133, 1942).
Root bark contains tannin, phlobaphenes and oxy-anthraquinone substances (Indian, Med. Gaz. 211, 1941): pulp contains rhein, the major anthraquinone derivative, small amount of volatile oil, three waxy substances and a resinous substance (Indian J. Pharm, 63, 1952).
Ayurveda : Aragvadha is said to cure haematemesis pururitus, leucoderma ascites and diabetes.
Distribution : Throughout India.

9. 'Samudrapalaka' (Vrddhadaraka) *Argyreia* speciosa Sweet Syn : Lettsomia nervosa Roxb (Convolvulaceae).

Roots are alternative, useful in rheumatism and diseases of nervous system.

Leaves emolent, poultices for wounds.

Chemistry : Fatty oil (J. Indian Chem. Soc. 83, 1947).
Ayurveda : Vrddhadaru improves digestion, gives clean complexion and cures diabetes.
Distribution : Throughout India, near sea shores.

10. Babuchi : *Psoralea corylifolia* Linn. (Leguminosae).

Seeds are used as stomachic deobstruent, diuretic and diaphroetic.

Chemistry : Seeds yield essential oil and psoralen (J. Indian Chem. Soc. 41, 1933), seeds contain resin, essential oil, a terpenoid oil, psorlen and isopsoralen (Proc. Indian, Acad, Sci, 5A, 351, 1937), psoralidin (J. Sci. Industri, Res. 28 B, 1948).
Pharmacology : Psoralen and isopsoralen possess the curative action in Leucoderma (Indian J. Pharm, 105, 1943).

Ayurveda : Seeds cure haematemesis, leprosy, leucoderma and diabetes.
Distribution : Throughout India, in dry places.

11. Ardraka : (Zingiber officinale Rosc.). (Zingiberaceae).

Rhizomes used in dyspepsia, flatulence, colic and other stomach diseases.
Chemistry : Rhizomes contain potassium oxalate (Pharm. J. Trans 802, 1892), 0.8% essential oil, camphene, B-phellandrene and Zingiberene (Curr. Sci. 322, 1945). Rhizomes yield 1 to 3% volatile oil containing comphene, phellandrene, cineol, citral borneol, and zingiberene; gingerol and shogal are the pungent constitutents (I.P.C. 256).
Ayurveda : Bhavaprakasa states it cures enlargement of abdomen (ascites etc) consumption, anemia, diabetes, allied diseases with excess urine.

12. "Bala": *Sida acuta* Burm (Malvaceae).
Chemistry : B-Sitosterol, A-Triacontanol and semi-solid ksteroidal matter, isolated; Glucose, fructose, glycosides and flavoroids found.
Ayurveda : In Bhavaprakasa it is recorded that "Bala" root bark powder with milk if (taken internally stops polyuria, while Mababala (*Sida rhombifolia* Linn) cures discontinuous urine discharge, correct `vata'. It also, if taken with milk, cures urinary diseases like Diabetes mellitus etc. and correct flow of urine.
Distribution : Throughout the hotter parts of India.

13. "Saptrangi" *Salacia prinoides* DC. and *Salacia macrosperma* wight (Hippocrataceae).

Decoction of powder stem and leaves are given to cure Diabetes mellitus.
Chemistry : Leaves, stems and root were isolated pre-anthocyanidin and quinones. Leaves yielded polyisoprene gutta and lecopelargonidin. (Curr. Sci. 34 : 634, 1965).
Pharmacology : Positive hypoglycemic activity (J. Pharm Sci. 56, 1405, 1967).
Distribution : In semi-evergreen forests of Western Ghats and Deccan.

14. Durva Dubh : *Cynodon dactylon* (Linn) Pers. (Gramineae).

In Ayurvedic this herb practically is taken as very sacred, very useful for urinary troubles, epilepsy and insanity.

Chemistry : Plant extracts contain alkaloids, and phenolic compounds.

Pharmacology : Shows potentiating effects of phenobarbitone, induces sleep, diuretic and possesses hypoglycemic effect. Aqueous extract shows reduction in blood sugar level (Neutral fractions).

Ayurveda : The fresh juice is said to possess demulcent astringent diuretic and haemostatic effects in case of cuts and wounds. Fresh juice is used in dropsy, chronic diarrhoea and dysentry.

Distribution : Throughout India.

15. Punarnava (Sant) : *Boerhaavia diffusa* Linn *B. repens*Linn. (Nyctaginaceae).

Roots of this herb are used in urinary affections.

Chemistry : Roots contain active constituent alkaloid, punarnavine, total alkaloid contents of roots, 0.94% (Indian med. Gaz. 204, 1923); Proc. nat. Acad. Sci. India, 240. 1934-35).

Pharmacology : Intra venous injections of the alkaloids in cats produce a distinct and persistent rise of blood pressure and marked diuresis.

Ayurveda : Cures are urinary infections and disorders.

Distribution : Throughout India.

16. Kaladi, Kela : *Musa paradisiaca* Linn var. *sapientum* kuntze Syn. *M. sapientum* Linn (Mussaceae).

The unripe fruits of *Musa paradisiaca* Linn are found useful in diabetes when given in combination with other drugs.

The juice of the flowers is given in dysentry and the sap in hysteria and epilepsy.

Pharmacology : From flowers of different varieties of banana, hypoglycaemic principle have been isolated (Planta Medica 16, 43, 1968). Seeds are reported to possess anti-small pox effect. (Planta Medica 15, 416, 1967).

Ayurveda : Root and stem, used in blood and venerial diseases. Unripe fruit: Diabetes. Juice of flowers: in dysentry. Sap of stem: hysteria and epilepsy.

Ayurveda or Hindu system of Medicine is followed since centuries in India. There are many medical classics which give treatment of diseases, which are not understood even in the modern times. Charaka Samhita, Sushruta Samhita and Ashtanga Haridaya are too well known. Diagnosis, treatment etc. are unique. Healing of disorders follows the treatment. This system is, therefore, followed in the Indian sub-continent.

In this paper, the concept of the disease "Madhumeya" or Diabetes as understood by Hindu physicians, is given. Sixteen specific crude drug plants, frequently used as a cure for diabetes is mentioned. Details of active principles, pharmacology as per modern text and Ayurvedic uses are enumerated:

References

1. Ashtanga : 1939, *Ashtanga Haridaya,* Vag Bhatt Acharya, Nirnay Sagar Press, Bombay (New Edition).
2. Caraka : 1941, *Charaka Samhita,* Agnivesha N. Sagar Press, Bombay (Reprint).
3. Chopra, R.N. 1938, *Indigenous Drugs of India,* Calcutta.
4. Collier, B.N. 1971, Comparative study of diabetes knowledge among juvenite Diabetics and their parents. Diabetes : 20(1) , 51.
5. Dhanwantari, 1925 : *Dhanwantari Nighantu,* Anandashram Press Poona (Reprint).
6. Drash Allan, 1971 : Diabetes mellitus in childhood-A review Jour. Ped. 78 (6). 1919.
7. jarret, R.J. 1970 : Lessons of Epidemology of Diabetes. Brit. Med. Jr. 3. 270.
8. Pyke, D.A. 1970 : General treatment of Diabetes, Brit. Med. Jr. 3 : 268.
9. Sushruta Samhita, 1882 : Sushruta Samhita (Translation) S. Nirnaya Sagar Press, Bombay, (Reprint).
10. Bhishagratna, K.L. 1963 : The Sushruta Samhita, (English Translation), Varanasi.
11. Shastri, H. 1971 : Clarification of "Deha Dhatu" and "Pancha Bhutagni", Jour. Res. Indian Med. 5(2), 183.
12. Sharma, P.V. 1971 : Panel discussion on the Ayurvedic concept of urine formation and urinary disorders. Jour. Res. Indian Med. 5(2), 186.
13. Taylor, K.W. 1970 : Diabetes-underlaying biochemical lesions. Brit. Med. Jr. 3 : 267.
14. Watt, G. 1889 : Dictionary of the Economic products of India, Calcutta.

VIII

Some Ayurvedic Plants Showing Immunomodulating Activity

Introduction

Although the discovery, that microbial pathogens caused infections diseases, was a key element that stimulated the formulation of modern immunology-the origin of a theory of an active immune response actually arose from another discipline-Inflammation as a defensive, and a beneficial mechanism.

Elic Metchnikoff-a Russian embrylogist viewed inflammatory processes as being central for establishing organismal identity and the phagocyte as being responsible for harmonizing potentially discordant cellular elements during development.

In the mature organism, these same mechanisms would be used to protect the host's integrity and defend against pathogens.

Immune identity involves the inter play of various immunocytes, in interactive roles.

It is too well known, that medicinal plants were used to cure human illness but the exact mechanisms was not known. It was known that plant drugs offer resistance against infection by reestablishing body equilibrium and conditioning the body tissues.

An attempt is made to evaluate the restorative and rejuvenating power of herbs, which may be due to their action on the immune system which is responsible for the protection of the organism from extraneous substances and maintain homeostasis (cf. Bellante 1978).

The present study in an attempt to investigate the effect of certain medicinal herb widely used in Indian system of Medicine for the treatment of chronic infections and immunological disorders, on the immunesystem of experimental animals. Azathioprine was used as a standard control.

Material and Methods

(II) Experimental Animals

Swiss albino mice 8 to 10 weeks old reared in our animal house were used in all experiments. For graft rejection inbred mice was used.

(III) Sheep Red Blood Cells (SRBC)

Sheep blood collected in Alsever's solution was washed three times in large volumes of pyrogen-free sterile normal saline and adjusted to a concentration of 5 x 10^9/ml for immunization and challenge.

(IV) Delayed Type Hypersenstivity

Delayed type hypersensitivity response to SRBC was induced in mice by the method of Lagrange et al (1974) as described by Doherty (1981). Groups of 10 mice per treatment were immunized by injecting 20 ul of 5 x 10^9 SRBC/ml S.C. into the right foot pad.

The plants under study were collected freshy from Jawarlal Nehru ayurved garden, Pune. Their germ plasm was studied and selected species was subjected for investigation.

The herbs were dried, then powdered to 20# size. Complete TLC pattern was studied with its active principles present. The drug was extracted in a Soxhlet with 95% ethanol and solvent removed under reduced pressure.

Aqueous suspensions of the extracts suspended in 0.25% gum acacia were fed orally to mice with a metal feeder.

The dose did not show any overt toxicity and this was determined for each extract using the dose-response curve, used to estimate the oral LD_{50} in mice. (cf. Miller and Tainter 1944).

The control group of animal were given an equivalent volume of gum acacia vehicle.

After a week (i.e. exactly 7 days later) the thickness of the left hind-foot pad was measured using a Vernier Calliper (Oditest, OOT, H.C Kroeplin GmbH. -Schluechtein F.R.G) measuring to 0.01mm.

The mice were then injected of 20 ul of 5 x 10 SRBC/ml i.d. into the left hind foot pad (O time).

Foot thickness was measured again + 24 h and + 48 h, after this action. The difference between the pre and post action-foot thickness expressed in mm was taken as a measure of DTH. The extracts were fed orally (10 ml/kg) on days-1, 0 + 1 + 2 + 3.

(V) Humoral antibody response

Another group of 10 mice were immunized by injecting 20 ul of 5 x10 SRBC/ml sc. into the right hind-foot pad.

Seven days later they were challenged by injecting the same amount i.d. into left hind-foot pad.

The day of immunization is referred to as Day O.

Blood samples were collected from individual mice by retro-orbital puncture on Day +7 (before challenge), for primary antibody titre and on day +14 for secondary antibody titre. Antibody levels were determined by the haemagglutination technique described by Nelson and Mildenhall (1967).

Equal volumes of individual serum samples of each group were pooled to serial, two-fold dilutions of pooled serum samples made in 25 ul volumes of normal saline containing 0.1% bovine serum albumin (BSA-Saline) in V-bottomed Takasty micro-titration plates were added 25 ul of 0.1% suspension of SRBC in BSA-saline.

After mixing, the erythrocytes were allowed to settle at room temperature for 60 to 90 minutes until control wells showed an unequivocally negative pattern (small button). The value of the highest serum dilution causing visible haemagglutination was taken as the antibody titre. Each pooled serum sample was titrated in five parallel doubling dilutions and the men titre of these determinations was calculated. The extracts were fed orally (10 ml/kg) on days-1, 0, +1, +2, +3.

(VI) Skin Allograft Rejection

Fitted minute patches of homologous grafts of skin were transplanted in groups of 10 inbred mice according to the method of Billingham and Medawar (1951). Graft survival time was determined by daily observation, the criterion being epithelial survival. Extracts (10 ml/kg) were fed orally daily till graft rejection.

VII Phagocytic Response

Phagocytic activity of the reticulo-endothelial system (RES) was assessed according to the method of Hudson and Jay (1980).

A group of 10 mice each were injected 160 mg/kg i.v. with a 1% suspension of carbon particles (10 to 25 ul size) in gelatin 30 minutes after the oral (10 ml/kg) dose of each extract.

Blood samples were collected from the tip of the tail at different intervals after injection for measuring per cent transpaency spectro-photo-metrically, at a wavelength of 675 nm.(Urikon 810 spectrophotometer, Kontron Ltd., Switzerland) till the transparency equivalent to standard (original pre-injection blood sample) was obtained. The rate of carbon clearance phagocytic under K) was calculated from the slope of each time-concentration curve drawn by plotting (100-mean transmittance value) as ordinate on semiloganthmic paper against time as obsassa.

(VIII) Statistics

Following Dunnett (1964) method, data was analysed-using analysis of variance and Dunnett's test.

Observations

Data obtained are recorded in Tables I and II below :

Table 1: Plants Showing Immunomodulating Activity

Botanical Name & Family	*Part Use*	*Ayurvedic Use*	*Ethanol Extracts Yield (%)*	*LD_{50} mg/kg (95%) Conf. limit*
1. *Ocimum Sanctum* (Labiatae)	Leaves	Fevers, Cough/Cold	15%	4200
2. *Ocimum Gratissimum* (Labiatae)	Leaves	Bronchitis	16%	4100
3. *Azadirachta Indica* (Meliaceae)	Bark	Skin ailments, fever	12%	1525
4. *Aconitum Heterophyllum* (*Ranunculaceae*)	Rhizoma	Tonic	12.5%	1880
5. *Tinospora Cordifolia* (Menispermaceae)	Stem	Tonihepato-protective	25.0%	2650
6. *Tylopora asthmatica* (Asclepidoceae)	Leaves	Bronchitis Asthma	15.0%	350

contd. . .

Botanical Name & Family	Part Use	Ayurvedic Use	Ethanol Extracts Yield (%)	LD_{50} mg/kg (95%) Conf. limit
7. *Picrorhiza Kurroa* (Scrophularaceae)	Roots	Chronic dysentry	30.0%	1280
8. *Hemi desmus indica* (R. Br. (Ascelipiadoceae)	Roots	Rheumatism skin affections	18.5%	2500
9. *Holarhena anti Dysenteria* (Apocynoceae)	Seeds	Dysentry anthelminthic	12.0%	1250
10. *Zingiper offinale* (Zingiberaceae)	Rhizome	Digestive disorders dropsy	15.0%	1365
11. *Eupharbia prostrala* (Euphorbiaceae)	Herb	Asthma	12.5%	1250
12. *Musa sapientum* (Musoceae)	Fruits	Gastric Ulcer.	15.5%	1375
13. *Centella Asiatica* (Umbilliferae)	Leaves	Ulcer's hypertension	20.5%	16.57

Table 2 : Immunological Activity Profiles

Species	Dose mg/kg	DTH 24 h foot Swelling mm change	Antibody Litre Primary 7 days	Antibody Litre Secondary 14 days	Graft rejec-tion Time	Phagocy-tic Index
1. *Ocimum Sanctum*	100	0.85 ± 0.05 (-2.22)	332 ± 75	230 ± 25	11.30 ± 0.45	0.26 ±0.04
2. *Ocimum Gratissimum*	100	0.87 (±0.03	332 ± 76	230 ± 25	11.30 ± 0.4	0.26 ±0.04
3. *Azadirachta Indica*	100	0.86 (±0.02)	335 ± 72	320 ± 25	11.45 ± 0.5	0.23 ±0.03
4. *Aconitum Heterophyllum*	100	0.90 (±0.06)	283 ± 62	208 ± 66	11.30 ± 0.36	0.2 ±0.02
5. *Tinospora Cordifolio*	100	0.90 (±0.04)	256 ± 70	204 ± 31	11.54 ± 0.37	0.26 ±0.03
6. *Tylophora Asthmatica*	100	0.63 (±0.03)	76 ± 21	230 ± 25	16.90 ± 0.45	0.10 ±0.06
7. *Picrorhiza Kurroa*	100	0.55 (±0.02)	55 ± 20	200 ± 24	16.50 ± 0.43	0.12 ±0.05

contd. . .

Species	Dose mg/kg	DTH 24 h foot Swelling. mm change	Antibody Litre Primary 7 days	Secondary 14 days	Graft rejection Time	Phagocytic Index
8. *Hemi desmus Indicus*	100	0.58 (±0.03	62 ± 20	300 ± 29	16.66 ± 0.45	0.10 ±0.05
9. *Holarrhena antidysentrica*	100	0.91 (±0.06)	64 ± 17	204 ± 31	12.40 ± 0.21	0.30 ±0.06
10. *Zingiber Officinale*	100	0.85 (±0.05)	65 ± 16	208 ± 28	12.56 ± 0.23	0.30 ±0.05
11. *Euphorbia Prostrata*	100	0.65 (±0.01)	60 ± 15	110 ± 16	11.56 ± 0.11	0.20 ±0.01
12. *Centella Asiatica*	100	0.75 (±0.05)	85 ± 14	120 ± 16	11.92 ± 0.2	0.18 ±0.01

Results

It was found that (I)
Picrorhiza Kurroa increase the DTH (delayed type hypersensitivity) reaction by 80% while *Hemidesmus indicus, Tylophora indica, Zingiber officinale*, reduced it by 80%.
(II) *Picrorhiza Kurroa*, enhanced antibody synthesis. *Holarrhena anti dysenteria, Hemidesums indicus, Tylophora indica* inhibit the reasons. The effect was more pronounced on primary antibody production than secondary antibody production.
(III) The influence of plant extracts on T-Cell function in VIVO was also determined by their effect on allograft survival time as cell-medicated immunity which is known to be responsible for the rejection of foreign skin graft (Bellanti 1978).
(IV) *A conitum heterophyllum, Hemidesmus indicus and Tylophora indica.*
Significantly increased the survival time of skin grafts while pierorhiza rurroa hastened the graft rejection.
(V) The phagocytic activity of the (Phagocytic response) of the RES was measured by the rate of removal of gelatin-stabilized carbon particles from the blood stream.

Hemidesmus indicus appear to reduce the clearance rate whereas the other extracts appear to hasten it.

The maximum effect was obtained with Picororhiza Rurroa. The results obtained in the present in the present study indicates that Picrorhiza Rurroa. Azadirachta indica. Ocimum sanctun are potent immunostimulant. Stimulating both the specific and nonspecific immune mechanizms while *aconitum heterophyllum, Holarrhena anti-dysentrica, Zingiber officinals, Tylophora asthmatica* appears to enhance the phagocytic function and to inhibit the humoral component of the immune system.

Ocimum gratissimum,· Ocimum, Sanctum, Centella asiatica, Euphorbia prostrata, Tinospora cordifolia appear to improve the phagocytic activity without affecting the humoral or CMI, while *Hemidesmus indicus* clearly suppressed both the cell-mediated and humoral components of the immune system.

The above highly prised traditional Ayurvedic drugs are used either as ingredients in formulations designed as adaptogens or in treating chronic infections such as fever and immunological disorders such as asthma and rheumatism.

Atal (1985, Doherty (1981), Karnick (1977), Lagrange et (1974), Nelson et al (1967), Shivpur et al (1973), Singh et al (1984), Godhwanit et al (1988), Miyazawa et al (1988), J.M. Van der Nat et al (1987) et. The present study, crude ethanol extracts of these drugs have been found to influence several different functions of the immune system more-over, these findings suggest their use in a variety of other diseases susceptible to immuno modulation.

The observations will stimulate further investigations of the herbal drugs with a view to discovering newer immunomodulating agents from plant sources and lead to better and more effective drugs.

References

1. Godhwani, J.L: Godhwani, and D.S. Vyas (1988) *Ocimum Sanctum*-a preliminary study evaluating its immuno regulatory profile in albino rats. Jour. of Ethnopharmacology 24 (2, 3)-1993-198.
2. Miyazawa, T Murayama, N. Ooya, L.F. Wang, Y.C Tung, and N. Yamaguchi (1988); Immunomodulation by a unicellular green algae (*Chlorella Pyrenordosa*) in tumor bearing mice. Jour. of Ethnopharmacology 24, (2, 3).: 135-145.
3. J.M. Vander Nat, J.P.A.M. Klerx, H. Van Dijk, KTD de silva and R.P. Labadies (1987). Immunodulatory activity of an aqueous extract of *Azadirachta indica* stem bark. Jour. of Ethnopharmacology, Vol. 19 (2). 125-131.
4. Karnick C.R. (1977); Ethnobotanical Pharmacognostical and cultivation studies of Hemidesmus indicua R.Br. (Indian Sarsaparilla) *Herba Hungarica* 16; 7-16.

5. Karnick C.R. (1970); Some useful Crude-drug plants of Hindu system of Medicine Acta Phytotherapeutica 17; (10); 181-199.
6. Karnick C.R. and D.B. Horgay (1975); Studies on the Indian Medicinal Plants used in Ayurvedic System of Medicine Part I. Tylophora asthmatica W & A and Tylophora Dalzellii Hook 7. Herba Hungaric 14 (1) 5; 22.
7. Karnick C.R. and Mrs. M. Kulkarni (1990); Immunization against Bacterial and Viral Infections using Ayurvedic Herbal Medicines-A Clinical trial. Maharashtra Medical Journal 28 (7-8) 115-122.
8. Karnick C.R. (991); a clinical trial of composite herbal drus in the treatment of Diabetes mellitus Aryavaidyan 5 (1); 36-46.
9. Doherty N.S. (1981); Selected effect of immunosuppressive agents against the delayed hypersensitivity response and humoral response to sheep red blood cells in Mice. Agents Actions 11 : 237-242.
10. Dunnett, C.W. (1964); Test of significance or lack of significance between a control mean and several test means-Dunnett's test. Biometrics 20; 482-494.
11. Hudson L and Hay F.C. (1980); Practical Immunology, 2nd Edn. Blackwell Scientific Publication London 73-92.
12. Lagrange P.H., Mackaness G.B. and Miller T.E. (1974); Potentiation of T-Cell-mediated immunity by selective suppression of antibody formation with cyclo-phosphamide Jour. of Experimental Medicine 139; 1520-39.
13. Miller L.C. and Tainer M.L. (1944). Estimation of Ed_{50} and its error by means of logarithmic probit graph paper. *Proceedings of Society of Experimental Biology and Medicine* 57; 261-264.
14. Nelson D.A. and Milden Hall P. (1967); Studies on Cytophilic antibodies. *Austiralian Jour. Expt. Bio. and Med. Science* 15 : 133-130.
15. Singh B, Sharma M.L., Bupta D.K., Atal C.K. and Arya R.K. (1984); Protective effect of Tinospora cordifolia Miers on CArbon tetrachloride-induced hepatoloxicity. *Indian Jour. of Pharmacology* 16; 139-142.
16. Karnick C.R. (1970); Phytochemical Screening of some Medicinal plants used in Ayurvedic System of Medicine. Jour. of Research C.C.R.A. and S 2 (3); 364-383.
17. Karnick C.R. (1975); Phytochemical Investigations of some Tylophora species found in India. Planta Medica 27 (4); 333-336.

IX

Immunization Against Bacterial and Viral Infections Using Ayurvedic Plants

Introduction

Coverging evidence from immunology neurophysiology, neuro-endocrinology, pharmacology and psychology indicate that, like any other system functioning in the interests of homeostasis, the immune system is integrated with other physiological processes and is *thereby subject to regulation*, or modulation by the brain. For example, lesions of electrical stimulation of the hypothalamus results in alternation of humoral and cell mediated immunity (of Stein M. etal 1976).

Lesions of the anterior hypothalamus in particular, have been found to protect animals against lethal anaphylatic reactions.

Hypothalamic lesions suppress Arthus reactivity whereas hypothalamic stimulation enhances this *in Vivo measure* of hypersensitivity. It has also been found that lesions in the hypothalamus can reduce response to mitogonic and antigen stimulation and stimulation of the hypothalamus can enhance antibody responses.

The central role of the hypothalamus in regulating neuro endocrine neuro-transmitters in the modulation of immune responses, a role that since been documented by the findings that lymphocytes bear receptors for hormones and neuro-transmitter substances.

Experimentally induced and naturally occuring variations in hormonal state influence immuno-competence and *in Vitro* and *in Vivo* immune responses are affected by serotonergic (generally inhibitory) and catecholaminergic and cholinergic (generally stimulatory) interventions.

Conversely, antigenic stimulation (or more likely, the immune response to antigenic stimulation) elicits neuro-endocrine changes, including changes in the firing rate of neurons within the control-medical hypothalamus.

These, and other recent data providing morphological evidence for neural modulation of *in Vivo* immunological activity (Williams J.M. etal 1981), document the multiple connections between the brain and the immune system.

Hormones and neurotransmitter are endogenous substances regulated by the central nervous, that are directly or indirectly involved in process of adaptation (eg. responses to stages).

Although the immune system of capable of some auto-regulation, the adaptive functions of the immune system that are of ultimate concern take place within a constantly changing neuro-endocrine environment, that is sensitive to external events, including behavioral processes of adaptation.

There is, then, a neuro-anatomical and neurochemical basis for a behavioral modulation of immune function (of Stain etal 1976).

Stimulation of Immune System

(or Immune Modulation)

The normal flora of the GI tract-serve to stimulate the natural antibody.

The antigens of the microflora of GI tract are processed and presented by the special zed micro-fold epitholium of the Payers patches. This sensitizes antigen, sensitive cells present here and in related lymph nodes.

Lymphocytes that get activated in this manner and having IgC and IgM, receptors settle in organs of the systemic immune system. Lymphocytes with IgA receptors return to lamina propria and become activated as plasma cells with produces antibodies not only against these antigens, but also non-specific antibodies.

Hence, the oral immunization by using herbal decoction having a broad spectrum enhancer of host defence mechanisms was brought into play.

Ayurvedic Management of Microbes

(Kirmi-"Skusme") in Indian Medicine, we have-what is known as 'Doika' theory of diseases, according to which, any change in homeostatis makes an individual susceptile to various diseases. Virus are found in Human body, they are always latent and becomes activity only when homeostatis balance in disturbed. Indian Medicine deals never to irradiate the infection, but to restore the homeostasis which retard further growth, in this we trigger the defence mechanism of the body to tackle the situation successfully, i.e. we introduce herbal decoctions which has properties to tackle the areas of growing infections and to bring back the situation to restore homeostasis. India is rich in various medicinal plants, both well-known to cure viral and bactericidal infections. The method is quite different since we base our treatment on hololistic principles and we know that entire human system is governed by Vayu, Pitta and Kapha which is controlled by Jatar-Agni (Gastric enzymes) and the entire body parts and organs are covered by "Space System" wherein flows the gases (Vayu) which is/can be changed by Jatar Agni-this vayu reaches the exact position, where homeostasis has been disturbed and lateral Virus/Bacterial-colonies are developed in such a way, it retards their growth and thereby bring out normality in any given situation of outside infection of Virus/Bacteria/ir-nuclear changes with any abnormal cell growth.

Drug Plant Selection

Following drug plants (herbs) were selected having Immuno-stimulatory activity

Aspecies	Active Principle	Action
1. Astragalus membranceus	Astragalan (Polysaccharidge) of Astragalus.	Immuno-potentiating
2. Alluim sativum (bulb-liliaceae)	Diallyl thiosulfonate	Immuno potentiating
3. Andrographis paniculate (Acanthaceae	Andrographolide	Anti-bacterial dysentry & lepto-spirosis

(Contd....)

Aspecies	Active Principle	Action
4. Iphigenia indica (Rh3) Zingiberaceae)	Colchicini amide	Anti-cancer
5. Curcuma aromatica (Rh3) (Zingiberaceae)	Curcumol curdone	Anti-cancer
6. Indigofera tinctoria (Leguminosae)	Indirubin	Chronic myelocytic leukemia
7. Nim (Azadirchta indica)		Antibacterial, shows immunodulatory activity.
8. Cynodon dactylon		Antibacterial
9. Swertia chirate		Anti-viral immunodulatory activity
10. Ocimum sanctum		Anti-viral immunodulatory activity
11. Eclipta Alba		Anti-viral
12. Wedelea calendulaceae		Antiviral + Cordefolin
13. Boerahavia deffus		Antiviral + Cordefolin
14. Phyllanthus neruri	(cf. Parist + Beauquesne) (1938, Parist Moyse 1963)	Antiviral
15. Phyllanthus emblica		Antiviral

Hot water extract were taken out of individual drug plant and mixed together in equal proportion on a sugar syrup. The syrup was tested of 30 rats for LD 50 and found none of the drugs were toxic and 100% safe.

Dose: 3-5 ml dose was given to give each child of various age groups:

The study is based on 300 children out of which 215 suffered from pyogenic menungites, gastroecnteristes, Broncho-Pneumonea, menungomylogicals and dermal sunus. Carried ero Ayurvedic Research Centre and Hospital Jhansi, during the tenure of 5 years. The diagnosis of the disease was made on the basis of clinical examination, cerebospinal fluid fondings blood/stool examination X-rays etc. The available datas were analysed statistically to evaluate factors effecting the fatality and effects of unmunopotentiating action of some ayurvedic preparations. In certain cases T & B lymphocyte counts, delayed hyper sensitivity test using PPD. Skin test, etc. (cf. Talwar 1983).

Observations

The findings recorded are recorded on Tables below :

Table 1 : Age, distribution and Mortality

Groups	*Age*	*No. of Cases*	*Mortality*	*Causes*
(a)	0-1 year	75	45%	Phogenic
	0-1 month	10	85%	Memongitis
	1-6 months	30	45%	
	6-12 months	35	35%	Clastroenteristes
(b)	1-5 years	50	25%	Broncho-pneumonia
	5-Above	15	10%	Menongo mylocele.
		215		

Table 2 : Duration of Illness and Mortality

Duration (Days)	*No. of cases*	*Mortality (%)*
0-1	36	19.4
1-3	42	26.2
3-7	47	46.9
7 and Above	12	66.7
Total	137	35.8

$X^2 = 14.41$; d.f = 3, $P > 0.01$

Table 3 Nutritional Status * and Motrality

Nutritional Status	*No. of cases*	*Mortality (%)*
Normal nutrition (Mother's feed)	55	32.7
Grade I (Maluntrition)	42	35.7
Grade II (Malnutrition)	29	37.9
Grade III (Malnutrition)	11	45.5

$X^2 = 0.76$, d.f = 3, $P > 0.05$.

Table 4 : Associated Illnes* and Mortality

Associated Illness	*No. of cases*	*Mortality (%)*
Absent	85	32.6
Prenent	51	41.2

$X^2 = 1.04$, d.f = 1, P> 0.05.

Conditions			
	One illness	38	Children
	Two illness	13	Children
	Illness UTRI	17	Children
	Skin infection	16	Children
	C.S.O.M.	14	Children
	Gastroenterites	8	
	Bronchopneumonia	6	Children
	Monongomylocela	2	Children
	Derma Sinus	1	Children

Table 5 : C.S. 7, Sugar, Leval and Mortality

C.S. 7 Sugar (mg/dl)	*No. of cases*	*Mortality (%)*
++ 10	78	44.9
10-40	51	25.5
40-Above	8	12.5

$X^2 = 7.08$, d.f = 2, P > 0.05.

Table 6 :

Age	*Prior Mortality (%)*	*After unmunopotentiating action of Ayurvedic preparation/Mortality (%)*
6-12 Months	20	5
1-5 Years	15	2
5-Above	12	2

Table 7 : Recovery Rates

Cases : 150 Children	*Slow (%)*	*Faster (%)*	*Recovery (%)*
6-12 Months	3	10	35
1-5 Years	5	15	35
5-Above	3	20	45

X = 14.41; d.f = 3, P > 0.01.

Results

Ayurvedic Medicinal Plants have been used to cure human illness since time immemorial. There are certain of these drug plants are said to promote normal health and maintain organic resistance against infection by re-establishing body equilibrum and conditioning the body tissues (Bhagvan Dash 1978, Savnur 1950).

Ayurvedic on its medical ethics have clearly indicated that there is a restorative and rejuvenating power of these herbal remedies could be due to their action on the immune system which is responsible for the protection of the organism from extraneous substances and maintaining homostasis (Bellanti, 1978). The word "Immune-System" was never used in Ayurvedic System of Medicine but they point out body resistance is built up by changing of homors i.e. Vate, Pitta and Kapha and thereby treating chronic infections and immunological disorders, on the immune of human beings.

We carried out animal studies wherever and TH (delayed type hyper sensitivity test); Humoral antibody response, phagocytic response LD 50 tests were carried out before using the herbal decoction on babies.

We found, Picrohiza Kurroa showed potent immuno-stimulant action, stimulating both cell-mediated and humoral activities on animals; while Tylophora asthamatieu Aconitum hetero phyllum, and Holarrhena antidysenterica stimulated phagocytic function. ON the otherhand. Tinospora cordifolia, qamum gratissimum improved the phagocytic function.

These Ayurvedic herbs in formulations are so designed as to as a daptogens, and treat chronic infections, as fever, and immunological disorders as bronchial infections and effect CNS of the growing child.

We further found that the mortality rates of Children was reduced whether it was yastro-enteristic, pyogenic menugites, Bronchial Pneumonia etc or mortality due to malnutrition etc.

References

1. Atal, C.K. (1985): Role of some important Ayurvedic Drugs in modulating the unimune system in the human body.
Indian Drug Manufacturer's Association Bulletin 16 : 17

2. Atal C.K : M.L. Sharma, A. Kaul and A. Khajuria (1986) : Immunology II W.B. Saunders Co. Philadelphia P.A. pp. 225-242.
3. Bellante J.A. (1978) : Immunology II W.B. Saunders Co. Philadelphia P.A. pp. 225-242.
4. Bhagwan das V (1978) : Fundamentals of Ayurvedic Medicine Bansal and Company Delhi India pp. IX-XVI.
5. Billingham R.E. and Medawar P.B. (951) : The technique of free skin grafling in mammals.
Jour. Exp. Bio 28 : 385-402.
6. Doherty N.S (1981): Selected effect of immunosuppressive agents against the delayed hypersensitivity response and humoral response to sheep red blood cells in mice. Agents Actions 11 : 237-242.
7. Dunnett C.W. (1964) : Test of Significance or lack of Significance between a control mean and several test means-dunnett's test. Biometrics 20; 482-494.
8. Hudson L & Hay 7.C (1980) : Practical Immunology 2nd Edn. Blackwell Scientific Publication London UK. pp. 73-92.
9. Karnick C.R. (1977) : Ethanobotanical, Pharmacognostical and cultivation studies of *Hemidesmus* Indicus, R.Br.
Indian Sarsaparilla. Herba. Hungarica 16, 7-16.
10. Karnick C.R. (1987) : Phytochemical Screening of some Medicinal Plants used on Ayurvedic System of Medicine. C.C.R & S Bulletin Vol. 2 (3); 364-388).
11. Karnick C.R. (1970) : Some useful Crude-drug plants of the Hindu System of Medicine. Acta Phytothera peutica XVII (10) p. 181-184.
12. Karnick C.R. (1978) : Responses of Lunarphases on the growth *Abrus Precatorices* Linn. (Legumunosae) and its effects as crude drug on diseases Acta Horticulturae 73. Spices and Medicinal Plants 239-247.
13. Khory R.N. and Katrak N.N. (1984) : Materia Medica of India and their Therpeutics.
14. Lagrange P.H., Mackaness G.B. and Miller T.E. (1974) : Potentiation of T-cell-mediated immunity by selective suppression of antibody formulation with Cyclo-Phosphamide. Jour. Exp. Medi 139 : 1529-1539.
15. Nelson D.A. and Milden Hall P (1967) : Studies on cytophilic antibodies Australian Jour. Exp. Bio and Medical Science 45; 113-130.
16. Savnur H.V. (1950) : A handbook of Ayurvedic Materia Medica, with Principles of Pharmacology and Therapeutics. Dr. Jaghast and Sons, Belgaum. India PP XX-XXI.
17. Shivpuri D.N. Singhal S.C. and Prakash Da (1973) : Treatment of Asthma with an alcoholic extract of Tylophora indica-A cross over-dpuble-blund study. Annals of Allergy 30 : 87.
18. Singhani B, Sharma M.L. Gupta D.K. Atal, C.K. and Arya R.K. (1984) : Protective effect of Tinospora cordifoli Micer's on carbon tetrachloride induced hepatotoxicity Indian Journal of Pharmacology 16; 139-142.
19. PietroDe Camilli and Francesca Navone (1984) : Immunocyto Chemistry as a tool in the study of neuro-transmetter actions. Vol. 5; P 300-303.
20. Nestler E and Greengard P (1983) : Nature (London); 305; 383-388.
21. Kennedy M (1983) : Annv. Rev. Neurosci 6, 493-525.

X

Indian Medicinal Plants Used in Management of Tumors (Cancers)

Body built in Mechanism

For several years physicians have known that, body is protected by a mysterious natural defence system that acts in the blood to seek out and destroy the army of germs that daily invade our bodies. Since time immemorable Hindu Physicians have known that they can mobilize the body's defence system and make a person immune to a disease. Same was rediscovered by 19th Century Doctors-that immunity to disease can be done by vaccinating etc. him, with a small amount of the germs of that disease.

Despite the well-known successes of this vacination principle in such old infections diseases as measles, diphtherea, small-pox, polio and now even veneral disease, immunology as a science languished in the masty book sections of the modern bacteriology laboratory.

Scients were wondering how immunity worked, to use it against other kind of killer disease.

Status of Immunology in Hindu Era

Cancer is now ranked as one of the fore-most killer in various parts of highly industrialised nations.

In Ayurveda, it is recorded that all disease of prolonged nature have their origin in Elimentary Canal, Stomach and its subsidary canals are interlinked by a unique glandular system which in return are controlled by brain. The disturbance in mental equilibrium effects these internal glandular system which passes its responses to stomach or any variation or disturbance in gases and other exchange lead to brain responses, may be adverse or otherwise. This could be set a-right by yogic exercise, intake of certain vegetable drugs which build the entire immune system and the disease was cured or even warded off. Master-gland according to them is pineal body of the brain and which can be vitalised by nerve compleses of the notochord.

Modern Status

Scientists have recently traced the immune system through the body, pin-pointing, that the thymus, a small gland near the heart, as the master gland, that controls one component of the body's immune-response, while, the bone-marrow as controlling the other components. As a result of these new understanding of the immune system, scientists have been able to tie immunity into almost every branch of medicine and have found it, to be in some cases immediately useful, and potentially promising in many more, as a weapon against disease.

Antibodies and Antigens

Two German chemists of 1890's who, having inherited the knowledge of vaccination from the early work of Louis Pasteur and the great Microbe Hunters in England, France and Germany, were on to tackle systematically the nature of immunity.

They discovered, there was actually a *factor in the blood*, a protein molecule, that chemically fights invading germs. This was subsequently called as *antibody* and the *invader* was given the name of the antigen.

Today we are in dark about different antibodies, the body can make, but it is now estimated that there are not less than tens of thousands of which the scientists relise that, each antibody is specifically designed to ferret out, i.e. fight and kill the particular antigen. While, the molecular structure of the antibody and how it is driven to recognize and fight germs is still, under study, in quite a large number of laboratories while entirely different approaches to the immune response were taking place elsewhere.

There was a report by Dr. Ogden Burton that a young patient, suffering unduly from various infections whose blood had no gamma glabulin-the blood protein out of which most antibodies are made. This was first report as on *Immuno deficiency disease* and it struck Dr. Robert Good of Memorial Sloan-Kettering Cancer Centre, New York, who had found that, when blood contain no gamma globulin, could not produce antibodies. There was one graduate student in poultry science at Ohio State University named Bruce Glick. He was studying out cropping of the chicken intenstine known as the *Bursa* of *Fabricus*. He found when bursa was large, the chicken grew into plump young foul. Later, it was found that bursa was evidently essential to antibody production and to immunity.

Immune Systems

The observations was, that chicken also has a thymus, which on the basis of Dr. Good's own observations, was lead expected to regulate the immune system.

This lead Dr. Good and Dr. Miller in England, to remove thymus from born animals to see that happens. Dr. Good recalls to say that "It dawned on me suddenly that chickens might have two immune systems and called it Two-component system".

There are two populations of immunity agents. Both arise out of basic steam-cell in the bone marrow and after undergoing changes are sent as lymphocytes or white cells into the blood stream, (Red cells are also made by the bone marrow, but serve only to carry oxygen and other substances to the organs and tissues). One population of white cells is knows as the T-Cells, because they mature in the thymus, the other population of white cells directly from the marrow without passing through the thymus and are called B-Cells, after bursa of the chicken. About 90% of the white cells are T-Cells and 20% are B-Cells. Interestingly enough, no other species, including man, has a burse in the muscles that are associated with bursitis).

The two immune-system operate in happy togetherness in the body, but have different structure and perform different duties. The bald billiard ball-looking T-Cells, sometimes called killer cells, are genetically programmed to search out and destroy the big preys. They go after skin-grafts, transplants, massive foreign bodies, even cancers, which they kill by virtually surrending them and clobbering them to death; on occasions they even penetrate the foreign cells. The hairy, tentacled B-Cells are more complex biological units, that do their job by sending forth the antibodies that combine with and kill the smaller antigens.

Each intruder triggers only, one kind of anti-body, which is designated to do. Recent experiment show, however, that for most infections, both sets of cells participate in immune response, possible through some chemical interaction. T-Cells tackle smaller preys, alongwith B-Cells, and B-Cells participate in some of the bigger kills.

The marvelous property of the system is its ability to recognize the cells of its own body as friends or as "self" and distinguish them from enemy cells or "Nonself" an ability to sensitively refined its amounts to what one investigator cells "Biological-fail-safe mechanism".

A New Medical Tool for Attack on Cancer

The first major clinical investigation to expand the knowledge of immune-response occured in 1967, when a small boy suffering a series of infections was examined by Dr. William Cleveland in Miami Florida. The doctor found that the boy had no thymus and no T-Cells in his blood, a disease known as Di-George Syndrome. Here was a case, that could show whether the patients defective immune-system could be manipulated medically, by reconstituting his blood with new T-Cells. Dr. Cleveland could get from a culture of thymus from aborted fetuses, a tiny thymos, no bigger than the end of a fingernail and injected the material into the infact abdominal muscle. Within 24 hours his lympocyts count began to climb. Four weeks later he could reject skin grafts. His blood showed an ample supply of T-Cells. Now seven years later, the child's dual immunity system is perfectly normal. Cancer is also suspected to be an immunological disease. There are now well-documented cases of cancers that disappeared as musteriously as they had come, especially when the patient came down with a *curable secondary infection* during the bout with cancer. Recently, for instance, a patient with stomach cancer developed peritonitis, an infection of the abdominal wall, this was cured and the cancer disappeared with it.

Aged people who immune-system less resilient than those of the young develop cancer at a higher rate than young people.

Children with immune-deficiency disease contact cancer at a rate of 100 to 1000 times greater than the normal population of children of that age. All of is suggests that the lack of immune response *encourages cancer* and vice versa.

A singular observation recently made, showed the possible role of the immune system in cancer treatment. This observation was made when patient who underweight, kidney transplants were found to have received organs that had tomors in them unknown to the do. When the doctor treated a transplanted patient with immune-suppressive drugs to prevent rejection, the tumor emerged and spread. As soon as the drug was stopped, the immune-system went back to work and the patient rejected the kidney alongwith the cancer. This observation clearly pointed to the envolvement of the immune system in cancer. It was also possible to establish that the T-Cells functions as the body's first line of defence against, tumors and that a *thymic deficiency* makes the body unable the cope with the disease.

In view of this increasing body of evidence, showing the relation between the immune-system and cancer. Doctors today are giving a lot of thought to methods that would tune up the entire immune-system of the body to make it as effective as possible against all invaders. Such a broad approach might help in destroying the antigens of cancer.

Experiments were carried into France, by Dr. Georges Mathew and his associates with a strain of bacillus known as *Bacillus Calmette-Gurein* (or B.C.G) which had long used as a tuberclosis vaccine and injected it into children dying of leukemia. His first clinical trial of this adjuvant, as such a booster vaccine is called, resulted in 1964 in a good response.

Subsequently he improved on the procedure by combining the B.C.G. with tumor cells from other patients and injecting them together. B.C.G., he believed, would raise the immunological level of the body and enhance the body's normal response to weak antigen's associated with foreign tumor cells.

Mathe claims that this synergistic arrangement produced longer survival times, among patients suffering from this form of cancer, but, scribes agent, whether the results arise from the immunity-agent itself, or from the kinds of patient selected for the tests.

Skin Cancer

Another form of immune-therapy useful mainly to treat skin cancer arises from attempts to take-advantage of body's delayed hypersensitivity to some foreign substances, a kind of allergic reaction in which the skin breaks out in a rash and itch.

Dr. Edmund Klein of Rosewell Part Memorial Institute in Buffalo, New York, who had been searching for a chemical substance that would cure cancer of the skin.

His experiments showed that one of the test substances caused allergic reactions that were more intense around the site of the tumor that elsewhere. Afterward, the tumor would swell, dry up and disappear.

Dr. Klein investigated various irritating chemical substances that produced hypersensitivity and found that some cases he could immunologically cure Cancer without seriously harming the patient. He now claims that 95 percent of his epidermal skin Cancer Patients have been permanently curved.

Others, with tumors have also been helped, but at a lesser rate of success. "The chemical substance itself has nothing to do with creating immunity to the tumor cells says Dr. Klein, "but it is simply a way to manipulate the delayed hypersensitivity of the immune-response to work for the patient".

Dr. Karl and Ingergard Hellstrom of the University of Washington in Settle, found that their exists a "Blocking factor", a complex antigen and antibody which appears in the blood of cancer patients, just as the cancer takes a turn for the worse. The substance is not detectable in the blood stream of patients whose tumor have regressed or stabilized. Hellstroms were hopeful of isolating, from patients, who are cured of cancer, an antidote that can be used in new patients to counter the blocking factor and allow the stymied system to go, to work, to kill the cancer. (Lec. Edson 1974 : The American Review 18 (4) : 28-36).

Ayurvedic Parameters

Cancer is a biological disturbance, a disease of more probably, a group of diseases, which affects all types of living beings, man animals and plants.

Cancer is the development of a new growth, a nodule or a tumor in the tissues of their origin.

Tumor is usually hard and firm to feel, which gets fixed to the surrounding tissues and is not movable in them.

The other characteristic of cancer is that the original tumor has a remarkable tendency to form colonies (secondary tomor's or metastases), in the same or distant parts of the body.

In a part of the body belaboured by blows from fits etc, the afflicted flesh produces a swelling.—17.

In a person fond of eating meat or whose tissues are vitiated, the swelling progressively increases in size. It is painless, greasy, uniform color, non-suppurating, hard-like a stone and not movable. This is Marsarbuda and it is said to be incurable—18.

In the (tumors, which appear) curable, the flowing should not be selected (for treatment). Those which have spread to vital regions, and those which if they are fixed and have arisen in srotas (Channels, e.g.-mouth, eyes, ears etc.).

A tumor originating in an already existing growth is designated as Adhyarbuds by Arbudednas (Tumor expers).

Tumor's which arise (in different parts of the body) at the same time or those which arise one after another are:

Dwirarbudas (Secondary tumors) and are incurable—20.

Indian Herbals Used

1. Tylophora indica — Entire herb.
2. Aloe vera — Leaves.
3. Glycyrrhiza glabra — Roots.
4. Emplica offcinalis — Fruits.
5. Hemidesmus indicus — Roots.

The above Indian medicinal plants were found to be useful in the cure of tumors.

Generally hot water decoctions were found to be useful. Dosage is governed by the severity of case and the age of the indurdual and his/her neuro psychological conditions.

Table 1 :Clinical Observation-O.P.D (R.R.C. Jhansi)

Sr.No	Disease*	No. of Patients			Partial/None
		Male	Female	Relief	
01.	Stomach Ulcers	10	8	16	2
02.	Stomach (Carcinoma)	2	1	1	22
03.	Tonque (Carcinoma)	8	—	4	2
04.	Cervissal (Carcinoma)	—	3	1	2
05.	Breast (Carcinoma)	—	2	1	1
06.	Throat	1	—	—	1

* Carcinoma : Hospital investigation. Treatment of all primary stages.

From the foregoing data and observations made it is observed that some of Indian herbal, do have a good potential in the cure of so-called "Carcinoma", whether it is immu-theraphy or cyto-enzymatic disturbance due to embalance of distray regime or factors controlling homors as per Ayurvedic principles.

Abnormality of vals, pitta and kapha are all interlinked with Jatar Agni which in turn depends upon type of food intake.

Recent observations have led us to believe that if certain vital glands which controls the internal secretions of the body are removed by surgery or destroyed by radiation, it brings about dramatic results in cases of advanced cancers of breasts in women and prostrate in elderly men.

This in line with Ayurvedic thinking that all internal secretions play a vital part in keeping with metabolic changes in the body and this depends upon type of food intake and vitiation of Jatarangni.

References

1. Cameron C.S. : 1956, The Truth about cancer, Prentice Hall, New Jersey.
2. Beren Blum I : 1952, Man against Cancer, The story of Research, John Hopkins Press, Baltimore 1952.
3. Oberling C : 1954, Le Cancer., H. Gallimard, Paris VII.
4. Ravew R.W. : Cancer Vols. 4-6, Batterworth, London, 1957-58.
5. Huxley J : Biological Aspects of Cancer, George Allen and Unwin, London 1958.
6. Greenstain J.P. and Haddow A : Advances in Cancer Research ols. 1-5, Avademic Press, New York 1953-58.

XI

Electromagnetic Effects on Human Tissue Systems

An understanding of the basic mechanisms involved in the interaction of electromagnetic fields with living systems can lead to an increased ability to provide healthcare, both from a research point of view and in terms of treatment.

It appears that non-linear mechanisms play an important role in tissue electromagnetic field interactions.

Non-linear molecular vibrations resembling soliton waves may be produced by externally applied fields, allowing for transport of energy released by chemical reaction at a distant site in long chain proteins such as enzymes.

Non-linear waves may couple reaction-diffusion processes, possibly both intracellular and extracellular.

Electrical Actions Along Cell-Membrane

One of the major unresolved issues in neurobiology is the mechanism by which ions move across an excitable membrane.

Hodgkin-Huxley model of membrane molecular action fails in the light of 29 years of research, which indicate on third or fourth order kinetics physically exist, as required by the model. Also, the model does not account for membrane excitability as a function of calcium. One can consider the cell-membrane as having a lipid bi-layer enclosed in a sandwich of structural protein, with external protrusions of glyco-protin whose strands terminate in negatively charged amino-sugars, (Adey 1977, Singer and Nicholso 1972).

These strands are the protrusions of intramembranous particles (IMPs). The IMPs are movable in the fluid mosaic of the lipid bi-layer. Contrary to the concepts of transductive coupling, some electrical events occur along the membrane in length and in area, rather than through the membrane in the transverse sense, as mostexcilatory processes have traditionally been viewed.

Superconducting Biological Josephson Junctions

The sensitivity of several organisms to very weak magnetic fields has led to the proposal that superconductive junction phenomenon may occur in these biological systems (Cope 1973). For example; experimental evidence is available for probable superconductive transitions in the cholates at temperatures close to room. (Wolf 1976, Wolf and Halpem 1976). Since water must be present in order to observe superconduction in the cholates, this suggests that they may be the "Sandwich" type of superconducting structure in which a thin film conductor is adjacent to the strong dielectric, so that electrons can propagate in the adjacent dielectric.

Biological system exhibit many such sandwich structure in which, layers of water are interfaced with protein and lipid charge conductors.

Also, weak magnetic field effects on probable Josephson junctions have been observed in carbon films of 25 deg. C (Antonozicz 1975), Josephson junctions between superconductive micro regions in living systems may provide a possible physical mechanism with more than enough sensitivity to explain the observed responses of organisms to weak magnetic fields. In addition microwave effects observed on probable room temperature Josephson junctions in carbon films suggest that non-thermal effects of microwaves in biological system may occur by the same mechanism (Antonowicz 1975) Cope, 1976 Antonowicz 1974).

Magnetic Neuro-muscular stimulation

Merton and Morton (1980) demonstrated single shock stimulation of the motor cortex through intact scalp and were able to induce motor contractor of the opposite limbs.

Barker and his colleagues in sheffield have stimulated 47 subjects, many times with no apparent adverse effects.

We have demonstrated this motor cortex stimulation and in addition have demonstrated phosphene production from visual cortex stimulation, peripheral muscular stimulation and deep pelvic and lumbor muscular contraction.

Depolarizing Nerve Cells

Action Potentials Generation

It has recently observed that time-varying magnetic fields could induce enough current within tissue to initiate depolarization of nerve cells sufficient to generate action potentials pulsed magnetic fields promote bone and soft tissue healing.

Antoine Priore of the French Academic des Sciences, France, was to cure thousands of cases terminal cancers and leukemias in Laboration animals.

Magnetic stimulation : —helps in recovery of paralysed bladder, diaphragm contraction.

Material and Method

Patients recorded in OPD, were selected and all clinical parameters, namely X-rays, Urine, Stools Tests were carried out. Nearly 300 patients, which were treated with electromagnetism (low level ELF modulated 350-450 MH3 fields).

Observations

Table 1 : (Various Age Groups, 18-60)

Symptoms	*No. of Patients*	*Response (Positive)*	*Improvement*	*Relief*
Fractures/bones	5	4 ± 1	4	4
Back-Ache	125	24 ± 1	23	22
Spondilysis	30	25 ± 2	24	24
Glandular Swelling	6	5 ± 1	4	3
Pelvic Pains	35	32 ± 2	30	32
Parlysed Bladder	5	6 ± 2	5	4
Pain in Stomach	75	64 ± 2	63	22
Peptic Ulcer	10	8 ± 2	6	4

Results and Discussions

The use of magnetic theraphy has been in vogue for over 5 years and over 300 patients have found relief and cure at various stages ailments.

The author with his team in his clinical trials observed that weak magnetic fields play a very significant role in getting relief to the patient, who have been heavily drugged with analgesic drugs with little relief.

Table I shows the data obtained substantiate the findings.

This chapter deals with electromagnetic effects on Human tissue systems. It appears that there is a positive interaction of electromagnetic fields on living organs, Non-linear waves couple with diffusion process brings about changes at intracellular and extra-cellular regions.

Electro-magnetism effects cell-membranes, the process is explained in details. Data shows that bone fractures, spondialysis, glandular swelling Odema, pelvic pains, etc. show definite response.

References

1. Davidson John (1989) : Subtle energy C.W. Daniel Co. Ltd Church Street, England.
2. Pearce, C.B. Ian (1983) : The Holistic approach of Cancer, A.N.A.C., Maidstone, England.
3. Reich W (1948) : The Cancer Biopathy, Orgone Institute Press, New York PP 97-108.
4. Grand B.R.J. Cadoret and G.I. Paul (1961) : "The influence of an unorthodox method of wound healing in mice" International Journal of Parapsychology 3: 5-24.
5. Becker Robert (1988) : U.S. Patent No. 4, 528, 265 Electrically generated ions can produce cellular activities and structural changes conducive to differentiation.

XII

Medicinal Plants having Anticonvulsant Activities.

Clinical Manifestations Classifications

Seizure's may be considered in three broad categories.

1. Focal, neocortical seizures.
2. Temporal lope seizures.
3. Primary subcortical seizures.

I. Focal Neocortical Type

(A) *Characteristics* : Aura-unconsciousness-tonic + clonic movements posticial drowsiness.
Electro-encephalo-graphic localization-Single or multiple cortical foci of spike's in any area of cortex.

(B) *Focal Motor* -Ayura-lateralized motor-cortical foci of spike's and slow waves.

(C) *Jacksonian*-March of motor events-cortical foci of spike's and slow waves.

(D) *Adversie*-turning of head side ways-frontal lobe origin.

(E) *Sensory* :

(1) Somatosensory-tingling, numbers-Partial lobe

(2) Visual-Flashing lights and colour, posticlal blindness (rare)-occipital lobe.

II. Temporal Lobe

A—Psychomotror and Emotional states-Automatisms, dream states, fear, and other emotional responses, lip smacking and chewing-Anterior temporal lobne foci.

B—Visceral and Autonomic-Epigastric, distress nausea, vomiting, sweating, tachycardia-mesial temporal foci.

C—Illusory and Hallucinatory-Olfactory (Unicinate fits). Sense of familarity (dejans) feeling of unreality, memory flahbacks formed visual hakkucinations-Mesial and anterior temporal foci.
D—Auditory and veriginous-unformed and formed auditory sensations, dizzness-Lateral temporal foci.

III. Sub-cortical

A. Minor Motor (Petitmal)-Brief lapses in contact with staring and speech arrest-Synchronous, symmetrical 3/sec. spike and wave disclvarg, no cortical localization.
B. Major Motor-Sudden loss of consciousness-Evidence of Synchronous firing from deep frontal regions.

Causes of Seizures

1. Severe Birth Trauma-Anoxia, confusion.
2. Congenital Maldevelopment.
3. Metabolic-Hypoglycemia, hypocalcemia, Hyponatrema, Urema, disorders of amino acid and vitamin metabolism, lipidoses.
4. Toxins and Withdrawals-Lead, alcohol, barbituratessss, steriods, organicphosphates, change in anti convulsants.

Material and Methods

Each capsule consisting of following herbal drugs namely :
1. Portulaca Oleracea Linn.
2. Nardostachys Jatamansi DC.
3. Allium Sativum Linn.

500 mg were used showing various types of seizures after taken narcotics like Bhang (Cannabis), or Datura eating of Mushroom (Wild). Phytochemical studies of each drug was carried out, TLC, HPTLC, Chromatography after taking alcoholic, Menthol extracts of drugs. Details investigations are recorded below:

Clinical evaluation of 30 patients were carried out Medical Research Unit at Ujjarin in Gwalior and Jatshi Medical College and Hospital. Results are recorded in Tables given below:

(1) *Portulaca Oleracea* Linn (Portulacaceae) : Parry O et al (1987); Jour. of Ethnopharmacology: 19; 247-253. An aqueous

extract of *Portulaca oleracea* effective in relieving muscular spasms—100 mg.

(2) *Nardostachys Jatamansi Dc* (Valareianaceae) Chemistry: Thizomes contain volatile essential oil (0.5%) (Oleum Jatamansi)- Ketonic principle jatamansone, sesquiterpene viz. seyhellene, seychelane and B-sitosterol. Roots norseychelanone, seychellen, patchouli alcohol and a and B-patchoulenese Oil-terpenic coumarains, oroselol, jatamansin-B-eudesmol, elemol, B-sitosterol anagelicin and jatamansinol.

Pharmacology: Antispasmodic, nerve sedative, useful of spasmmodic hystercal affections—100 mg.

Alluim Sativum Linn (Liliaceae) : (Agel et al 1991: Direct relaxant effect of garlic juice on smooth and cardiac muscles. Jour. Ethno-pharmacology 33 (1, 2), June/June 1991- (13-19). Garlic extract completely abolishes the spontaneous movements of rabbit jejunum and guinea pig ileum. It also inhibited the contractions of guinea pig tracheal smooth muscles.

Chemistry-Active principle of garlic-5-ally cysteine sulfoxide, crystallized from water acetone, Aminoacids—10 ml.

Observations

Formulation was based on Ayurvedic Medicine was prepared from the following drugs :

Table 1

S.No.	Local Name	Botanical Species	Part Used
1.	Foneka	Portulaca Oleracea Linn (Portulaceae)	Entire Herb
2.	Jatamansi	(Nardostachys Jatamansi Dc (Valerianaceae)	Roots
3.	Alluim	Sativum Linn (Lilacea)	Bulb (Oil)

Table 2

Patients	50
Age	49.5 ± 2.5%
Disease Duration	1.5 ± 0.5
Sex Ratio M/F	20/30
Body Weight (Kg)	58 ± 5.5

Wilcoxon and Studients "t"-test

Data expressed as mean ± S.W.M.

Table 3

S. No.	*Criteria*	*Symptoms*	*Drugs taken*	*Post treatment status*
1.	Focal Neocortical	dversive	*Mushroom* Sp	0.4 ± 0.15
2.	Temporal Lobe	Psychomotor & Emotional States	*Datura* Sp	1.5 ± 0.17
3.	Subcortical	Minor Motor (Petitmal)	*Bhang*	25. ± 0.19

Results : Out of 50 patients demographic and clinical data are recorded in Table III. Treatment of formulation controlled the regiours and seizuresto 32%. These who were taking drugs regularly for over an year were found too be partially incapable of doing work. Slight intake of Bhang or Datura effected their mental capacities, become lazy and could not do without it and become habitual narcotic takeres. The drug was found to give relief to patients and stopped continously heaving and regours.

References

Arisa T. Oshiba S and Tamada T (1981); Platelet aggregation inhibitor in garlic. *Lancet* 1 (8212); 150-151.

Van Breemen C (1971); calcium requirement for activation of intact sortic smooth muscle. *Jour. of Physiology*; 272; 317-329. Bhide V.P., Pand A, Sathe A.V., Rad V.G. and Patwardhan P.G. (1987) Fungi of Maharashtra *Govt. Press India*.

Zamora-Martincz, Mariselac and cecilia Nieto de pascual Pola (1992); Medicinal Plants used in some rural populations of Oaxaca, Puebla and Veracruz, Mexico. *Jour. of Ethnopharmacology* 35; 229-257.

XIII

Calotropis and Zingiber in Migraine Head-Ache

Introduction

Migraine is a recurring head-ache with an irregular interval. It may be classified as under:

(i) *Migraine head-ache*: Incidental head-ache accompanied by visual gastro-intestinal and or premenstrual disturbance.

(ii) *Cluster head-ache*: (Migranous peuralgia) episodic attacks of pain behind one eye, which becomes red and watery. Attacks occur once a day lasting between 20 to 120 min. for 6 to 8 weeks.

In both types of migraine, muscle construction (tension head-ache) unilateral or bilateral.

Dalessio (1980) Rose, (1985) has elaborated various causes for head-ache and other head pains, with advances in the knowledge of Migraine. There is now general agreement on the causes and the mechanism of Migraine.

Blau (1985) considers migraine as a neurological disorder with some evidence of the involvement of some vascular phenomenon (Dalessio, 1980).

We used two drug plant powders namely dried buds of *Calotropis procera* linn and dried rhizome of *Zingiber Officinale* Rose in exact propositions and founds the results were very promising. Out of 10 patients, 59% of them were completely free of pain within span of 3 to 7 days.

Material and Method

The author in his Tribal Survey of Tribal Medicine came across a unique method used by tribals to cure head-ache the plant they often use is buds of *Calotropis Procera*, R Br. to be taken with milk.

As per Ayurvedic principles-the cause of head-ache is vitiation of Vayu in Jatar Agni. This is usually corrected by Adrak or sunte (Zingiber Officinale).

Out of lab tribals led us to formulate a new combination using both drug plants and results were found very promising.

Patients having Arda-sisi (Half head) with long period of troubles were chosen. 10 such patients were chosen in our OPD and capsules prepared by us were used internally, early in the mornings by the patients, till pains last. Results are recorded in Tables given.

Table 1 Showing the Effect of Ayurvedic Drugs on Patients (Cast History)

S. No.	Age/ Sex	Condition before	Condition after use of Caps.
01.	35/M years	Migraine (right side) stomach, pains tension	Lessened pain within 2 days stomach pain disappeared, relaxed.
02.	25/F years	Head-ache for last 3 days after menses, red eyes	Head-ache stopped within 3 days. Menses cleared.
03.	27/F years	Pain in ears, one side head-ache nostrils filled feels vomiting.	Stopped nostril cleared. digestion improved, pain stopped relieved.
04.	40/M	Pain in ears, one side head-ache for last 2 weeks stomach pain.	Ringing of ear, Head-ache lessened stomach pain disppeared pain stopped after 3 days.
05.	10/M years	Half head-ache cannot concentrate in school studies vomiting-tension	Head-ache disapper after 3 days. Feels. Stooped releieved.
06.	12/F years	Half head-ache whole night feels uneasy vomiting	Head-ache disappeared after 5 days. Feeling of vomiting stopped.
07.	30/F years	Pre-menstrial trouble. continuous half head-ache uneasy vomiting.	Menses cleared. Head-ache stopped after 6 days. feeling better.
08.	40/M years	Half-head-ache since one and half month head injury	No change
09.	40/F years	Half head-ache Ear-ache	Slight change feeling better pain stopped after 10 days
10.	42/F	Half head ache Menses trouble leńcorrhoea back pains.	Relieved 10% slight pain, but bearable after 7 days.

Migraine in modern context-is related head-ache's and are a collection of pain syndromes involving blood vessels (Johnson 1987). Many of the agents in use in modern therapy in use for migraine is either modify the release of transmitters in pain transmission (Opiates, somatostatin and calcium antagonists) block snesitization of nerve fibres (serotenia and biatamine receptor antagonists, pre-sterodal anti-inflammations (NSAI) or block inflammatory. Mechanism involving the blood vessel wall (serotonin and histamine antagonists, NSAI).

Nanda et al (1980) found that anti-histaminergic agents like the cimetidine/mepyramine combination, have been to be effective in spontaneous migraine.

A new histamine (H2) antagonist has recently been patented for the treatment of vascular head-ache. (Young R.C. et al, European Patent No. 181163). Knman 1919-observed that powdered flowers of calotropis in small doses are useful in the treatment of colds, coughs, asthama and indigestion. It contains unidentified tetracyclic compounds and calcium oxalate. Latex contain proteo-elastic enzyme similar to papain (Wealth of India series Vol. II C).

Ginger (Gingiber officinale) contains anti-histamic and anti-oxodant factors. (Duke and Ayensie, 1985).

The role of free radicals as endogenous histamine releasers is recognised (Mannaione et al 1988).

Prostaglandin endoperoxide synthetase is known to be a source of free radical histamine liberators (Shivarajah et al 1978).

Ginger, reported anti-histamic properties could be related to its ability to inhibit the formation of free radicals from arachidonic acid and other compounds known to indice histamine release.

We found that ginger and calotropis inhibit strongly prostaglandin synthesis (Kiuchi et al 1982, Srivastava 1984 a). Some components isolated from ginger were found to be even stronger inhibitors of prostaglandin synthesis that indomethacin (Kiuchi et al 1982).

Ginger has been used in Ayurvedic and Unani systems of medicine for head-ache, nervous diseases, nausea and vomiting for hundred of years. These observations have withstood the tests and inquiry conducted with the help of modern biochemical and pharmacological techniques.

Mowery and Clayson (1982) demonstrated that the gastro intestinal symptoms of kinetosis were alleviated better by ginger than by anti-histamine agent or a placebo.

Grntved et al (1988) reported subsidence of symptoms of nausea and vertigo after powdered ginger root (Zingiber officinale) consumption in a double blind rendomized trial in motion sickness (Sea sickness).

Backon (1986 b) has suggested that possible use of ginger in several psychiatric problems where inhibition of thromboxane A2 is required.

References

Backon J : Carbon dioxide inhalation therapy for anxiety; Effectiveness due to increased prostacyclin and decreased thromboxane synthesis; Re-evaluation of the negleted technique *Medical Hypothesis* 20 : 351-356 (1986).

Backon J : Ginger inhibition of thromboxane synthesis and stimulation of prostacyclin; Relevance for medicine and psychiatry. *Medical Hypothesis* 20 : 271-278 (1986).

Blau J.N. : Migraine Pathogenesis : The neural hypothesis re-examined *Journal of Neurology, Neuro-Surgery and Psychiatry* 47, 437-442 (1984).

Blau J.N : Pathogenesis of migraine headache; Initiation Jour. *Royal College, Physicians of London*, 3, 166-168 91985).

Dalessio D.J. (Ed) : Wolff's headache and other head pains; *Oxford University Press*, New York (1980).

Duke J.A. & Ayensu, E.S. : Medicinal Plants of China *Michigan* P. 657 (1985).

Johnson, E.S., Kadam N.P. Hylands, D.M. and Hylands P.J. : Efficicacy of Fever few as Phophylactic treatment of Migraine, *British Medical Journal* 291; 569-573 (1985).

Johnson G : Recent advances in Migraine Research; *Annual Reports in Medicinal chemistry* 22; 41-50 (1987).

Joseph R Steiner, J.T. Poole, C.J.M., Littlewood, J. and Rose, F.C. : Thromboxane Synthase inhibition. Potential therapy in Migraine *Headache* 25; 204-207 (1985).

Kiuchi F, Shibuya M and Sankawa U : Inhibitors of Prostaglandin biosynthesis from ginger *Chemical and Pharmaceuticals Bulletin* 30, 754-757 (1982).

Mannaioni P.F., Giannella E, Palmerani B., Pistelli A Gambassi, F., Banni-Sacchi, T., Bianchi, s and Masini E. : Free raducals as endogenous histamine releasers *Agents-and Action* 23, 129-142 (1988).

Marone G, Sabotka A : and Lichtenstein LM : Possible role of Phospholipase A2 in triggering histamine secretions from Human basophiles in vitro *Clinical Immunology and Immuno-Pathology*, 20, 231-239 (1981).

Mowery D.B. : Motion, Sickness, Ginger and Psychophysics *Lancet* 655-657 (1982).

Nanda R.N., Arthur G.P., Johnson R.H. and Lambie E.G. : Cometidine in the propohylaxis of migraine; *Acta Neurologica Scandinavica* 62, 90-95 (1980).

Rose F.C. (Ed) : Migraine, Clinical and Research Advances, *Krager* Basal (1985).

Shiva-Rajah K, Andersen M.V. and Eling T.V. : Metabolism of Benzo(a) Pyrene to reactive intermediate(s) via Prostaglandin biosynthesis *Life Scechces* 23, 2571-2578 (1978).

Srivastava K.C. : Effects of aqueous extracts of onion, garlic and ginger on platelet aggregation and metabolism of arachidonic acid in the blood vascular system; in vitro study.

Prostaglandins leukitriences and Medicine, 13, 227-235 (1984 a).

Srivastava K.C. : Aqueous extracts of onion garlic and ginger inhibit platelet aggregating and alter arachidonic acid metabolism *Biochimica et Biomedica Acta*, 43, S. 335-s. 346 (1984 b).

Srivastava K.C. : Isolation and effects of some ginger components on platelet aggregations and eicosaniod biosynthesis.

Prostaglandins Leukotrienes and Medicine, 25, 1987-198 (1986).

Srivastava K.C. : Effect of Onion and Ginger consumption on plate-let thromboxane production in humans *prostaglandins Leukotrinnes and Essential Fatty Acids*, 35, 183-185 (1989).

Grntved A, Brask T Kambskard J and Hotzer E : Ginger root against sea sickness-A controlled trial on the open sea. *Acta Otolaryngologica* 105, 45-49 (1988).

Wyscocka-Babowska M.M. : in F.C Rose (Ed) Migraine, *Clinial and Research Advances* Krager, Basal, P. 244 (1985).

Young R.C., Smith I.R., Brown T.H. and Mitchel M.R. : *European Patent* No. 181163 (1985).